CONCENTRATION

A GUIDE TO MENTAL MASTERY

BY MOUNI SADHU

This book was written to bridge the gap between the many existing theoretical works on mental concentration and meditation, and the general application of the mind's powers to everyday life. Mouni Sadhu teaches concentration by showing the use and results of it. By means of his unique system, the reader can learn to control his own thoughts, get the utmost from his abilities, and shape his life into a reasonable and logical pattern.

After a careful explanation of the role of concentration in a spiritual search and some helpful advice on proper approach, the author introduces exercises in concentration. He offers material from both Western and Eastern sources, relating the achievements of early Christian saints and Indian yogis to their mastery of mental powers.

Prior knowledge of oriental terms and techniques is not necessary, and no unusual physical powers are needed. The practice can be conducted in a quiet spot at home or out of doors. No sudden change in personal habits is required, although the use of alcohol and large amounts of tobacco is likely to retard progress in concentration. Proper balance in amounts of food, sleep and work is recommended, while a positive attitude and the will to succeed are emphasized as essential to mental mastery. The ability to reason soundly is the foremost condition of success.

This unusual and inspiring book offers the reader practical experience of the higher states of consciousness. Both logical and mystical, *Concentration* is not limited to any particular system of philosophy and its techniques.

Bibliography.

By Mouni Sadhu

Concentration

In Days of Great Peace

18 17

Concentration

A GUIDE TO MENTAL MASTERY

Mouni Sadhu

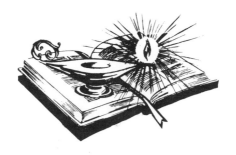

Melvin Powers
Wilshire Book Company

12015 Sherman Road, No. Hollywood, CA 91605

Sadhu, Mouni.

Concentration, a guide to mental mastery. New York,
Harper [1959]

222 p.   22 cm.

Includes bibliography.

1. Yoga.   ɪ. Title.

B132.Y6S32   181.45   59–6327 ‡

Library of Congress

ISBN 87980-023-2

To my unforgettable Guru
and his true disciples
this book is dedicated

BIBLIOGRAPHY

Besant, Annie, *Study of Consciousness,* Adyar, India.

Brandler-Pracht, Dr., *Geistige Erziehung (Spiritual Education)* (German), Leipzig, 1921.

Greek-Orthodox Scriptures, *Lives of Saints.*

James, William, *Variety of Religious Experiences,* 1899.

Leadbeater, Charles W., *Occult Talks,* Adyar, India.

Lodyschensky, P., *Mystic Trilogy* (Russian), Petersburg, 1912.

Maharshi, Sri Ramana, *Gospel,* Tiruvannamalai, S. India, 1946.

Ouspensky, P. D., *Ancient Tarot Cards* (Russian), Moscow, 1912.

Ramacharaka, Yogi, *The Inner Teachings of the Philosophies and Religions of India,* L. N. Fowler, London, 1918.

Ramacharaka, Yogi, *Rajah Yoga,* 1912.

Sadhu, Mouni, Two collections of essays, *Glimpses on the Path* and *In Search of Myself,* published between 1953–1957 in English, German, Brazilian, Indian and Japanese philosophical and initiatory periodicals.

Sadhu, Mouni, *In Days of Great Peace,* Bangalore, 1952 and G. Allen & Unwin, London, 1957.

Sankaracharya, *Viveka-Chudamani (The Crest Jewel of Wisdom)* (Translation by Mohini M. Chatterji), India, 1888.

Sédir, Paul, *Initiations* (French), Paris, 1922.

Sédir, Paul, *Quelques Amis de Dieu (Some Friends of God)* (French), Paris, 1923.

Vivekananda, Yogi, Various lectures and writings.

"Who" (Sri Lakshmana Sarma), *Maha Yoga,* Tiruvannamalai, 1948.

Wood, Ernest, *Concentration,* Adyar.

CONTENTS

7

P A R T   I I I
Techniques

P A R T   I V
Conclusion

PREFACE

This book has been written to bridge the gap between the many existing theoretical works on mental concentration and meditation, and the general application of the mind's powers to everyday life.

The extensive literature on these subjects provides plenty of "commandments" as to what should and should not be done and when to develop control of the mind. But it is not easy to find the most important and essential advice which concerns the practical answers to the unavoidable questions "How?" and "Why?"

More than half a century ago a gifted and experienced American—William Walker Atkinson, writing under the pen name of Yogi Ramacharaka, published a series of very useful books on Eastern philosophy and Yoga, which were wisely and purposefully based on his "Eclectic Method."

His main works are *Hatha Yoga, Raja Yoga, Gnani Yoga, Fourteen Lessons in Yogi Philosophy and Oriental Occultism,* and his final message under the title of *Philosophies and Religions of India.* These are perhaps the best of their kind and are unique, filled with practical advice.

He selected the best material he could find from the various known scriptures of his day, without any corresponding effort on the part of other contemporary occultists.

In the second half of this century, great advances have already been made in psychology in general as well as in occult psychology, and today we know far more about the human mind and its workings than did our forefathers.

Today, details may alter in the methods of dealing with man's main motive power—his mind; but the fulcrum of this present study remains unchanged.

The writer has impartially tried to collect in this book the best and most tested methods and exercises, plus all necessary explanations, which later may give the student a basis for his own deliberations, by revealing previously unperceived horizons. In particular, it is hoped that the exercises in Part III will serve this purpose.

This work may prove useful for two types of readers:

1. The near agnostic who wants to rule his mental powers for the improvement of his status and circumstances. For him, only portions of the book will be of interest, namely the practical exercises in Part III together with the explanatory chapters of Parts I and II. He has no need to go beyond the seven double exercises—Nos. 1 to 7A.

2. The seeker of things deeper than his own temporary physical appearance, who will find it necessary to study the book as a whole with special attention to the explanatory chapters in Parts I and II, and the culminating ones in Part IV treating the final conclusions of supermental achievement. This is *guided* intuitional knowledge, also called the wisdom of the Self, which is the ultimate aim of concentration.

In the beginning, no particular creed is required of either type of student. The ability to reason soundly is the foremost condition for success. Such an ability will be developed into a higher power of cognition by using, as a base, its sharpened tool—the perfectly controlled mind, which will then begin to reflect the reality of man's ultimate essence, the immortal and illimitable spirit.

This book is not limited to any particular system of philosophy and its techniques, and material has been freely drawn, according to its value, from both our Western and Eastern inheritance.

The author, throughout a lifetime of searching, has found that there are few things known to the highest circle of advanced Easterners which are not known to their Western counterparts, and vice versa, providing these men are earnest enough and endowed with the requisite abilities and qualities. The outer forms of the Eastern and Western traditions may differ, but not their innermost initiatory contents.

I

Foreword and Definitions

The Latin origin of the English word "concentration" has a clear and definite meaning. It refers to that which has a common center, or is moving toward a center, and is best expressed by the term "one-pointedness," which, etymologically, is not far from the literal sense of the Latin.

In this study I will try to show, in a purely practical way, how the human mind can be concentrated in order to gain the ability of one-pointedness. The necessary psychological and technical explanations will be kept to the minimum essential to enable the student to start his exercises with a reasonably clear understanding of what he is doing and why. *"Why, When and How should a study of concentration be undertaken?"* and *"What is to be attained if the study proves successful?"*

Imagine that you have an unsharpened pencil or a small stick. If you have to use either of them to pierce a piece of cardboard, you will find it difficult until the ends of your simple implements have been properly sharpened. Even considerable pressure exerted on an unsharpened pencil will not produce a neat hole. Why? Because a simple physical law is at work. Your power has been dissipated over the whole, comparatively large surface of the blunt instrument, thus providing

15

insufficient force to separate and remove the particles of cardboard and form a clean hole.

Similarly, a blunt knife or saw does not cut well and the result is unsatisfactory since the effort is wasted by being spread over too large an area and too many points. It is not concentrated.

But sharpen your tools and there will be no difficulty in piercing a hole or cutting a straight line. Where then lies the secret, if any? Merely in the fact that force applied through a single point acts more effectively and seems far greater than the same force simultaneously exerted on many points. This elementary law should be clearly and strongly established in the mind of anyone studying concentration. It is the justification for all the exercises that follow in Part III of this book.

Here we are not seeking to perfect a physical tool. The proper employment of the mind is our first aim—the mysterious power and attainment which can be gained only by use of a well-sharpened, one-pointed tool. With regard to the human mind we may call this the "thinking principle."

At this point I would like to quote from the sayings of the most recent of the great Indian rishis (or sages)—Sri Ramana Maharshi, who was an authority on occult psychology and all questions pertaining to the human mind:

"An average man's mind is filled with countless thoughts, and therefore each individual one is extremely weak. When, in place of these many useless thoughts, there appears only one, it is a power in itself and has a wide influence."

We know that many great scientists and inventors, whose ideas are now serving humanity, often ascribed their unique discoveries to just this capacity for strong, concentrated thinking. This was the case with Isaac Newton, Thomas Alva Edison, Louis Pasteur and many others, all of whom were conscious of and able to use their extraordinary powers of concentration, i.e., the ability to think solely about the object of their investigation to the exclusion of all else.

In Latin America, people who are unable to control their minds and forever wander from one thought to another are jokingly, but very appropriately, referred to as having *"quinhentos pensamentos"*—"five hundred thoughts"—at one time.

The idea of sharpening or concentrating our minds is neither new nor illogical, but rather scientific, since it has definite means and aims which can be thoroughly investigated, applied and reached.

II

The Method

Any secondhand treatment of this subject will be of little use to students who really want to get positive results from their efforts. So, in this book, I have systematically gathered together a number of practical exercises, all of which have been used and tested as regards their effectiveness.

Some of them may already be familiar to occultists who have long been engaged in the study of concentration. Some have been developed by the writer himself, while others were taken years ago from sources now no longer available, as the authors are long since dead and their books have disappeared. These latter exercises are the work of the most authoritative and competent exponents, but nevertheless they have all been chosen according to one standard—tested proof of their usefulness and safety.

The worst that can happen to a student lacking the will power to fulfill exactly all the instructions as prescribed, is nonattainment and no results.

This will undoubtedly be the lot of anyone who attempts to reap the fruits of concentration purely for his own egoistic and material aims; for concentration is not the final target. It is only a necessary ability and tool which allows a man a higher and better level of life-consciousness, otherwise unattainable by laymen in this particular subdivision of occult training.

The method adopted here is based on a strict grading of sequence of the student's steps. The exercises themselves have been limited in number to the absolutely indispensable minimum. This is very important, as every change gives rise to some fluctuations within the mind, and this should be avoided as far as possible. But not even the smallest detail should be omitted from the exercises, because the success of the endeavor depends upon the exactness of their application.

The beginner may know nothing at all about the method facing him and he is strongly advised *not to read in advance* any of the chapters beyond those on which he is working, especially the advanced ones (Chapter XVIII and XIX), until all the preceding ones have been mastered. This will be your first small showdown with the rebellious and selfish mind. There are very many instances where people have spoiled their work and extinguished their enthusiasm by unnecessary curiosity, which is only harmful and destructive.

Why not ask your mind here and now, *"Which of you is boss?"*

Instead of concentrating the mind, reading in advance will only create additional burdens to distract an earnest student who is working for really positive results. And there are quite enough obstacles to overcome and troubles to avoid without adding to them. Curiosity is the true creator of problems and by yielding to that vice how can we expect to acquire the opposite virtue, which is peace of mind?

This does not mean that we should completely abandon thinking with our present, more or less developed minds. That would be ridiculous and is not at all what I mean. What we are fighting for in this work is our inner freedom and balance, and the inescapable—but how welcome—mysterious, inner, but most real knowledge. It is the fulcrum on which will rest your whole inner world, and this is the *only thing* which a man can take with him into Eternity, no matter in what forms or worlds he may continue to manifest himself. It is essential that you curb the excessive curiosity of your mind for at least the short periods when you are working for perennial instead of mortal and ephemeral things. Do you not agree that these half-hours or so should be free from the slavery in which you are at present held by your uncontrolled and unruly mind? Its conquest will yield you something which, once gained, may end all the deeper questions of your life.

III

The Use of Concentration

The power of concentrated thinking as applied to everyday life is very well known and widely recognized. It does not need any proof or special explanation. But the average man does not use even a fraction of that power properly. If the reader disagrees with this, then I would like him to explain to me, or better to himself, if he knows *why* he is thinking in a particular way and not in another. Why some thoughts come to him, no matter whether or not he "invited" them. And if he can foretell what things he will be thinking about a few minutes hence. Can he really of his own will close his mind to an annoying or obsessing thought? Where do his thoughts actually come from?

If these questions remain unanswered, then we have to recognize that we are not masters of our minds. To put an end to this far from desirable condition is one of the first and foremost aims of this study of concentration.

Control of a machine means that we are able to put it into action, modify its speed and finally to stop it when needed. This is just what is required of a disciplined mind.

True concentration is not merely an ability to direct and maintain our *full* and *exclusive* attention for some minutes on,

21

say, a pinhead; but rather it is the ability to stop the thinking machine and look at it when it has ceased revolving. A craftsman feels sure that his hands will obey him and execute the exact movements he requires. Indeed, he does not even think about it and works without worrying whether or not his hands will do just what he wants at a given moment. Under such conditions hands and other human organs, when working properly, constitute a harmonious unit, capable of functioning in their own particular sphere of action.

Imagine now that some part of your body refuses to obey the impulses issued from the control center of your brain. For example, instead of pouring a glass of water when you are thirsty, your hand lights a cigarette or even refuses to move at all. Surely you will consider that such a hand is of little use.

Now look closely at the functions of your mind-brain. Can you affirm with utter certainty that you always think only when and about what you really want to, and that therefore you know from where your thoughts and feelings come into the light of your consciousness? Can you withhold the entry or limit the duration of thoughts in your mind for as long as you wish? If you are able to analyze your thinking processes, your honest answer will be in the negative.

So it would seem that the average man is not a good craftsman, because he cannot control his chief tool—the mind and its thoughts. His life is spent in using and accepting something which originates outside his reach and understanding.

The practical study of concentration opens to us the world not only of results, but also of causes, and lifts us beyond the slavery of uncontrolled feelings and thoughts.

An amazing example illustrating the direct influence of concentrated human will power on matter is that of a needle turning in a glass of water. Mme. H. P. Blavatsky used this to train her disciple, Mrs. Annie Besant, and to test the results of that training in concentration.

Place a small needle in a glass of water and to prevent it sinking, cover with a thin layer of grease by smearing your fingers with a little oil or butter and passing the needle between them. It should then be lowered carefully and slowly onto the surface of the water so that it floats freely in the middle without touching the sides of the glass.

Sit facing the glass with your chin cupped in your palms, elbows supporting them and resting on top of a table. Then when the needle is lying quietly on the surface, gaze at it intently with a strong desire to turn it by the sheer force of your will, concentrating on it as if imaginary beams were issuing from both your eyes. Do not blink. According to every rule of concentration, no other thought should be permitted to enter your mind and all your attention must be focused on compelling the needle to change its position by about 45 to 90 degrees. Breathe slowly and rhythmically as this may accelerate the result. If your concentration has been strong enough, the needle will gradually start to turn as desired. Later on, the process may become much faster, as your experience grows and with it your will power.

In some occult schools, especially those of Tibet, there is much importance attached to this exercise. However, in this course I wish to speak plainly about things without adding unnecessary trimmings. The exercise has its value because it is relatively easy to understand and perform and is a visible test of acquired ability. If well performed, it may give the student much self-confidence and faith in his powers, apart from incontestable proof of the possibility of influencing matter by the direct concentration of the human will, with all its possible consequences, which the student can investigate and realize for himself.

Perhaps it would be better to try this exercise after some closer acquaintance with others described in Part III. For example, it could be used in conjunction with No. 4A in Chapter XIX. Then you will be more likely to succeed.

The student must not talk about his exercises, and this applies to all the techniques given in this book. Do not discuss your project with anyone, except perhaps those who are known to you to be following the same line of work. But absolute silence is still preferable.

Talking only wastes your will power and greatly impedes the success of the exercises. Moreover, the curious thoughts of those who know about your efforts will persecute you and only add to the burden of unwanted thoughts you are trying to destroy. It will be enough if you *know* this and observe silence, thereby avoiding disappointment.

IV

The Role of Concentration in a Spiritual Search

In the West, we usually refer to those who are performing such a search as saints, mystics and spiritually minded seekers; while in the East they are termed yogis, sadhus and sannyasins. If we carefully analyze their lives and methods of attainment, we will undoubtedly recognize that the one thing which distinguishes them from average men is their conscious, one-pointed and intensely concentrated lives, wholly dedicated to an idea, which they believe to be their highest.

Saints and yogis gain control of themselves by steady practice. When one of them is immersed in his prayers and pious meditations, he has achieved that state only because he possesses a certain degree of domination over his mind and feelings. His only tool is his power of concentration, although it may still be far from perfect. Often such a man may even be unconscious of the name which we are using here to define his ability. With a yogi, that is usually not the case, because as a rule he is fairly conscious of his tools, and often possesses an elaborate set of theories which he uses to follow his particular path. Such a man, as the reader may recognize, is a living proof of the fact that concentration is essential to yogic practices. The particular ways in which an Eastern seeker applies his power of concentration do not matter as far as this study is concerned.

While the saint repeats his prayers day and night, the yogi will do the same with his mantras, pranic currents or mental images. The tool always remains the same, although under different names. In this book, things will be spoken of from a nonsectarian and impartial point of view, which does not involve the student in accepting or rejecting any particular creed.

For those who have been fortunate enough to see a man belonging to one of these types of "seekers" there must be the recognition that their first impression of him was that of an inwardly, deeply concentrated man, and not of a helmless boat tossed in all direction by the waves of the unconquered mind and its children—thoughts.

Now we should turn our attention to another very important factor in a spiritual search, also based on the one-pointedness of the mind. It is the power of concentration which can be, and so often is, used in the form of what we call prayer. What is true prayer? Nowadays the word itself is often misused and misinterpreted. The so-called "elite" circles of a number of occult and mystical organizations are far too quick at comparing and identifying prayer with different forms of their favorite modern term—"meditation."

Some people who are negatively disposed toward prayer often attempt to justify their attitude by offering the following sort of reason to the general public: The conception of prayer is ridiculous to every serious thinker, for it implies that when someone prays about anything, hints and advice are being given to the Almighty on how He should act, and what He may bestow on the worshiper. Such a conception deprives God of His most sublime qualities—omniscience, absolute goodness and love of humanity.

Unfortunately, too many people of mediocre intelligence readily accept such treacherous and senseless statements.

We will now try to show the depth of ignorance hidden behind this misnamed "scientific" point of view.

Such an opinion is based on a childish concept which has long since been rejected by all enlightened seekers of Truth, for it supports the greatest of all fallacies: that God is a person and is something separate from the life created by Him; that our relationship to Him is like that of opposite poles or the two sides of a coin, i.e., two things which are forever different.

If it were true that God and His creatures possessed such characteristics, then these quasi-philosophers might be right; but if the matter is carefully studied, the cardinal error in such a judgment will be easily seen.

We are not something separated from the Whole which we call God. Our consciousness is a fragment of His consciousness, no matter how infinitesimal it may appear to us at first sight. Our life, which is just this living consciousness, is a reflection of His life as the Whole.

Every true philosophy teaches, and great religions reveal to us, that He is omnipresent, for there is no place in the universe from which He is absent. And that we live only in Him, since we can never exist apart from Him.

These facts change things completely.

That which prays is not a foreign and separate entity worshiping some far-off lord of the world. No! It is a ray of the light of the same Absolute, which asks of its source and not of some cruel deity, and which pays homage to the same central infinite Light. It is apparently (but only apparently) a temporary and finite being.

Such a being, proceeding directly from the central consciousness, does surely participate (although perhaps unconsciously) in the creation and perpetuation of the manifestation of the unmanifested Absolute.

And such a being has every right to worship with the hope that its prayers may be heard and fulfilled.

Analyzing the process of prayer, we will find that there are different kinds and degrees of it, more or less perfect and pure, and therefore more or less effective.

Man's consciousness is able to merge into and become one with the consciousness of the Whole, i.e., God.

One person may pray about material advantages, another about the welfare of his closest relatives or for the relief of sickness and so on. This level corresponds to the more commonly known, but primitive types of "meditation" in some occult schools and similar organizations. Such meditations have as aims, elevated or ecstatic ideas, visualizations, development of definite virtues, etc., all of which belong to the realm of the mind, i.e., the highest manifestation of consciousness in the average man as we know it.

The thinking process linked with the emotions is the common basis of such prayers and meditations and is just what we may see around us every day.

On this level, prayer may have some advantage over the corresponding type of meditation, for in it appears an important factor—a degree of devotion to the Highest Being, which is often lacking in the "meditations" so beloved by occultists and similar people.

There is no power on this level more purifying than devotion. The heart of one capable of feeling it is always nobler than that of those who are considerably more mentally developed, but who lack this vital quality.

In the chronicles (diaries and biographies) of exceptionally advanced human beings, we usually find that an utterly different kind of prayer was used by these great saints of both the East and West. There were no requests for earthly benefits, no thoughts and, perhaps, no emotions in the everyday meaning; but just this mute, mysterious spiritual prayer so well known to the first Fathers of the Christian faith and to the later great followers of the Teacher Himself, like St. Francis of Assisi, St.

Vincent, St. Jean de Vianney of France (who lived only a century ago) and many others unknown to the general public, like St. Seraphim of Sarov in East Russia (eighteenth century), and so on.

When we are able to approach such a sublime form of prayer, then we may be able to understand why the highest type of meditation by far transcends those appearing in books, and is very close to the ideal prayer-meditation, as shown by the great Rishi Ramana Maharshi when he says:

> Perfect attainment is simply worship, and worship is attainment. . . . You should worship the Highest by giving up your *whole self* to *Him* and showing that every thought, every action, is only a working of the *One Life (God).* . . .
> —*Instructions to F. H. Humphreys*

What an example of concentration!

This highest form is beyond all thoughts, mental images, words and emotions. In it, the primordial light—which once created life as we know it—is reached, and nothing more remains to be attained.

In the works of that great contemporary mystic and disciple of a true master, the late Paul Sédir of France who died in 1926, we may find many scientific descriptions of this exalted form of prayer, for he was fortunate enough to be able to practice such worship. In explaining the question of the so-called unchangeable destiny of man, his master once told him:

> The imminent future can be modified by the conscious efforts of enlightened people, which take the form of prayer. As there is no "personal decision of God" there cannot be any irrevocable "decisions" at all, for who would make them?
> The manifestation of the universal life is like the ever-moving currents of a river. The waves are constantly changing shape and even the river itself may alter the lay of its bed.

Therefore there cannot be any so-called unavoidable fate or destiny, inflexible and inexorable. The living consciousness—God—cannot be subjected to such limitations, and who could impose them?

If God is the only possible, and hence self-contained, existence, embracing all and everything, penetrating the wholeness of manifestation like the ether of the ancient philosophers, then His reflections and rays must of necessity participate in Him. And so the power of prayer coming from His devotees is part of His own illimitable powers.

The Maharshi, substituting for the word "God" his own term "self" tells us that "there is nothing apart from or beyond that self." And Sankaracharya says: "In truth, this whole universe is only Spirit."

Christ spoke even more definitely when He stated: "I said you are God's." Giving us the idea of the fatherhood of God, the great Teacher defines our relation to the Highest as that of children to their parent, and not as "things" created for the temporary pleasure of a cruel deity.

So the prayer of a child is a different matter from that of a creature begging from a far-off dispenser of good and evil, as some would-be philosophers like to imagine.

Now we can better understand from whence comes the enormous power of prayer, so often noted, not only by saints but also by many average men. We can find many striking examples in contemporary literature where prayer has helped in situations which quite logically—from the standpoint of human foresight and possibilities—have appeared to be hopeless.

The higher forms of meditation lead on to the superconsciousness of Samadhi. The ecstasies of Western saints who used prayer are akin to these same states of consciousness. If the famous *Imitation of Christ* by Thomas à Kempis is studied, it will be seen that yogis do not possess a monopoly of the state of Samadhi. Knowledge derived from countries of differing culture and traditions often has an exotic appeal which excites our curiosity, but frequently proves to have been well known long ago in our own countries under different names and forms.

The wise old Ben-Akiba stated truly when he said: "All this was before and long ago; there is absolutely nothing new in this world."

In true prayer there is another factor which is lacking in the lower forms of popular meditation. And it is the surrender—even for a short time—to the Highest.

What is really meant by even a modest and imperfect surrender to the Lord? It is the surrender of what one believes to be himself, i.e., his triple manifestation, mortal and finite—body, emotions and thoughts, the two latter being his "soul" according to accepted theory.

Is this wrong? By no means! For even by a temporary surrender of the unreal part of him, a man already—even if unconsciously—recognizes the existence of the higher principle in himself. And this is undoubtedly progress for a man.

There are infinitely more people who are better able to pray than to meditate. For them, prayer is something much closer and understandable, as well as instinctively far more natural. The Maharshi said: "What is not natural is not permanent and what is not permanent is not worth striving after."

Those who are acquainted with the higher aspects of meditation always prefer its snowy peaks and the magnificent, incomparable view of Infinity seen from those heights. And those who approach the Infinite Lord by their devotion, devoid of egoism and greed, will also find what they are seeking. Perhaps they may meet in that mystical land of attainment, as, for instance, the great saint who reached Wisdom through love, and the great sage who attained perfect Love through his wisdom.

Just as a falling drop merges into the ocean, so each will lose his separate existence and be absorbed into the motionless sea of Perfection.

V

Who Is Qualified to Study Concentration?

Usually the first answer to suggest itself is "he who knows what he wants." In other words, the student must have a definite aim, and for its attainment he must realize that the foremost condition is the ability to concentrate. Mere interest, curiosity or other petty motives can never be factors leading to success.

Aims may differ, unless one is engaged in a true spiritual search, but all of them should be soundly based and not impracticable. Among the many I would like to mention only a few examples:

The desire to shape one's life into a reasonable and logical pattern; to get the utmost from one's abilities; to acquire peace of mind; to develop the art of avoiding outer suggestions as regards one's way of thought; the development of a strong will to enable one to steer one's life into any chosen channel.

If the student has only petty aims, such as: the ambition to develop some psychic abilities for the performance of so-called occult tricks in order to influence and puzzle others; to profit materially from the exhibition of his powers; to suggest to others that they do something against their convictions and

32

will, and so on—then it would be better for him not to try at all, because the result will be contrary to what he expects. Not a strengthening, but a considerable weakening of his powers will be the ultimate attainment in such a case.

Everything which is unreasonable and unjustified by strict logic should be avoided if you are to reap the best results from the exercises you will find in the following chapters. (See Part III, Chapters XV–XX.)

If you commit something which you know—through cold and impartial analysis—to be unreasonable and unnecessary, then factors foreign to your true self are at work in you. Then *you* are not the one directing your life, but are rather a slave of powers which are not exactly known to you. In religious terminology they are referred to as temptations, passions, and often as sins. To succumb to all these things indicates an extremely weak will power in a man. But concentration is in itself proof of a more developed will power. These two are opposite poles—weakness and strength.

It is a psychological law in man that the greatest inner strength can be generated only by pure and sound inspiration, and by a will well armed against passions, lower desires, fears, uncertainty and hypocrisy, and independent and free from any outer compulsion.

For without this will factor no study of concentration and successful achievement of the target is ever possible. Now you may see the sequence and interdependence of things which seem to form a closed curve, or a circle.

The wise person uses this knowledge as his guide, while the fool merely tries to free himself from the circle, from which there can be no escape.

All of the aforesaid should be well considered and thoroughly realized if you wish to qualify for an earnest study of the subject of this book. Concentration cannot be a refuge for weaklings, or an escape from well-earned karma, or as a means of gaining something, despite that karma which affects the three lower worlds of the physical, the astral and the mental.

Another explanation may be even better: to pass successfully all tests on the complete techniques of concentration and the accompanying practical philosophy, may be far harder than gaining a university degree. Although many normal men and women are capable of satisfactorily completing a degree course, *not* all of these same people are able *to create in themselves something which was not present before,* namely, the ability to concentrate instead of just acquiring a load of mental baggage.

Of course, I am not attempting to present concentration as a panacea for everything and everyone. It would be illogical, if not nonsensical; for, as in the case of the innumerable painters throughout history, not every one of them could have become a Raphael or a Rembrandt.

The idea of inner control and its performances is *true* and *fruitful,* but only for those who are able to *see* it.

There must be an inner attraction to the art of concentration and not just the expectancy of repulsive work.

Now the answer to the question expressed in the title of this chapter—"Who Is Qualified . . . ?"—should come more easily to you. Having read this chapter, you are in a position to analyze and decide for yourself whether or not you are ripe enough. But do not forget the other side of the coin: if *your heart* tells you to do it—obey its voice.

VI

Conditions for Success

There are some physical conditions which to a certain extent might influence the success or failure of your efforts to study this book. Of course, there are usually exceptional cases in everything, but they do not affect the general rule. I will mention just a few of these conditions.

1. An extreme physical weakness, resulting from disease or an ailment, and which affects your will power, is a clear obstacle to any inner effort by a beginner. For example: a man may say, "I realize the necessity of perfecting my thinking apparatus and will power, but my physical limitations are hindering me from beginning what I recognize to be very useful." Such a person cannot have much hope of following our way.

2. Too many heavy engagements in everyday life, which leave no time or energy for systematic and continuous practice. For such a person a weekend's concentration with all its exercises will be almost useless.

3. Lack of inner, intuitional and firm conviction that work of this kind will actually open for the individual the gateway to a new and better life; for there cannot be any compulsion in a study as subtle as this. Under such conditions a man should abandon the whole enterprise as being too premature.

On the other hand, if you completely agree with what you have read in Chapter III ("The Use of Concentration") and if you are able to arrange the few preliminaries given as preparation in Part III, then you may act with reasonable hope of full success.

The right psychological condition is that of recognition that you are not your mind, which should be your servant and not your master. This has been beautifully expressed by H. P. Blavatsky: "Mind is a good servant, but a cruel master."

Also, you should know that the way of concentration leads much further than to the mere capacity for one-pointedness of mind. Actual success means nothing less than the understanding of the mind's nature and source, and the simultaneous transcending of both these factors. It is the entering into a new state of consciousness about which you cannot possibly know or anticipate anything until you achieve the twofold realization just mentioned.

As a rule, the conditions for a fruitful study spontaneously arise for those ripe enough for the purpose.

It is worth mentioning that the idea will not present itself if the possibility does not exist for the enlargement of consciousness in this way.

One has ears and eyes, it is true, but one *must* be able to hear and see through these organs, which is not possible for everyone. Christ told us plainly that there are people who have ears and eyes, but yet who hear not and see not.

There must also be a firm decision in these matters, for, once disappointed, the student does not easily, if ever, return to the same studies. Doubts arise in him, and as he is still weak (the very fact of hesitancy is proof of this) he cannot resist the whisperings of his own mind, which tell him to abandon the whole idea.

It will be well if you accept even in theory—what is for many of us a fact—that *the mind is inimical to every effort on the part of man to subdue it.* This is because this subtle form of energy has its own dimmed consciousness which is not always identical with that of a man's. Too often the interests of both—man and his mind—are opposed.

You can observe the following simple example for yourself: Often when you need to use your mind-brain, it refuses to co-operate and finds many excuses such as fatigue, lack of time, anxiety, etc. The writer, at any rate, was helped greatly by developing the idea of separateness between man and his mind, in addition to the fact that his spiritual master had affirmed that such a division is useful and corresponds closely to the actual truth.

VII

Advice to the Student

Some people have a wrong idea about the methods and outcome of a study of concentration. And often some of them
cherish the belief that the very fact of belonging to different
occult and initiatory organizations puts them in a better position to grasp the ripe fruit of success, which they imagine will
fall into their hands without too much effort on their part.
Surely, they are still as far from their misty aims as they were
at the beginning of their strivings.

I myself have seen gentlemen performing different exercises
taken from books of a purely theoretical character, while re-
clining in easy chairs and puffing smoke rings from their ciga-
rettes. Similarly with ladies knitting away peacefully, perhaps
at underwear for their grandchildren. I do not know how far
this type of person can advance.

We should realize that the ability to concentrate—which,
considered practically, is the root of all the higher abilities in
a man—is quite serious and strenuous work, calling for the
whole of our attention and not just a few minutes each day,
the results of which may be quickly forgotten or submerged in
our busy daily round. It is much harder than earning a degree,
as I mentioned previously, and it is not a matter of filling one's

mind with the thoughts of others from books and trying to solve and answer problems and questions already solved and answered long ago.

Concentration is very different from that. The average man is usually born without this ability, at least to a degree worthy of mention. So he usually passes through life. But in this line of study you have to change your former nature and create something which was not present before. It is quite a different problem from that of learning the formal concepts of, say, philosophy from books and lectures.

An example may be helpful: When you matriculate, many professional courses are open to you. You may become a doctor, professor, lawyer, clergyman or what you will. But you make your choice because you feel that one particular profession and its studies and no other is best suited to you. Some simply say that they love their chosen work. Exactly the same thing must happen to you when you decide to study concentration. Everything will go well if you begin the exercises in Part III with *pleasure and keen interest*. It will not be of much use trying to perform them if they are an annoying and unpleasant task. This should be well understood before a start is made.

The effort to master concentration is a long-distance journey. In the first place, it will give you no tangible advantage or gain, and no degrees or honors. So somewhere deep inside you there must be something which inspires you to such an apparently abstruse study.

Some will say, of course, that if and when success does come, you will easily obtain practical benefits like those mentioned in the previous paragraph. Yes! But will you then care about titles and visible honors?

Concentration will not necessarily cure your physical diseases or change your personal karma. On the other hand, if the study is successfully conducted to the end, its final aim, the complete domination of the mind, will give you the key to the new consciousness which opens the mysterious gate from which you can see your life as it really is. Then you will recognize that even the unchanged karma belonging to your petty personality is something really *apart* from you.

If you think deeply about what you have just read, you may find its real meaning. It is not advisable to give anyone a "ready-made" truth. Things must be discovered and tried personally, just as no one else can eat and digest food for you in order to give you the necessary strength to live.

As you will see for yourself, the first two parts of this book are really an introduction, explanation and preparation for Part III, which is composed of the actual exercises and techniques. This has been done deliberately in order to help the earnest student first to lay a solid basis for his work and to understand why, how and under which conditions he may study concentration and what he may expect from it. It is essential to create your own clear, individual conception about the foregoing remarks so that knowledge may take the place of your former uncertainty and anxiety.

On psychological grounds, continuous self-examination (which is a consequence of the anxiety and restlessness of the mind) as to whether or not you are progressing quickly enough, is a great hindrance to concentration. It robs you of quiet self-confidence which is a vital condition for success.

When you have attained some advanced degree of domination of your mind by the newly gained ability of one-pointedness, you will see that your best progress was made when you *quietly performed the exercises* without worrying about the mistakes made or how many steps ahead yet remained.

Realize that the essential thing in concentration is your actual work along the line chosen and not just the empty deliberations of your mind.

Later you will also see that the greatest enlightenment, inner peace and joy come to you when your feverish thinking is reduced to a minimum.

So why continue to do *now* something which you know to be an obstacle that must be removed before success can come? A religious man will say that this is a state of affairs which involves a certain kind of "faith." This may be so, but a label means less than, say, the really good contents of a wine bottle. But then, what of a full bottle without any label . . . ?

PART II

Psychological Preliminaries and Keys

VIII

Eastern Methods or Yoga
(Mind before Heart)

Nowadays, when we speak about concentration and other occult practices, the Eastern tradition or Yoga often comes involuntarily to mind. But the methods of inner progress and acquisition of subtle powers (and, as the crown of them all, the realization of man's true being or self) have their followers in countries outside of India and other exotic Eastern lands.

The West possesses its own particular methods and exercises which lead ultimately to the same unique goal.

From the many existing branches of Yoga we will examine only those which use concentration as their motive power. We may find a perfect parallel to our own study in the mental Yoga called Raja Yoga (i.e., Royal Yoga). Its object is to attain perfect control of the mind which then sometimes acquires what to laymen are wonderful qualities and powers. On these are based all the tricks and phenomena of the lowest type of Indian occultists such as fakirs and others, many of whom are not even occultists but are merely more or less able showmen.

Anyway, in Raja Yoga the mind and its functions are put before another power in man which is often called the heart. From the start we hear little about feelings and emotions, apart

45

from constant admonitions that both must be dominated and removed from the field of consciousness of a Raja yogi. This happens because of an assumption that if the mind, as superior to the emotional counterpart in man, has been subdued, the lower one—also called the "astral body"—will automatically be controlled. This may be so at times, but not always. Before you become a yogi, an advanced occultist or a saint, the astral body (feelings) and mental body (thoughts) in your everyday consciousness are practically *indivisible*. And this side of things is often overlooked by second-class teachers of Yoga. The proof? Yes! we have it. For example, do you know why there sometimes arises in you a particular feeling which has a stream of thoughts as a direct consequence? Or why, when certain thoughts occur, they bring with them particular emotions and remembrances of feelings?

It is very hard for an untrained beginner to penetrate into the origin of the currents in his consciousness. But as Raja Yoga insists, we should start with the mind first. Here a very accurate conception is put forward—you and your mind are not identical. This is quite a logical statement. Otherwise, how could a teacher of Yoga train you to dominate your mind if both you and he were the same as your minds?

You will also hear another important statement, with which, however, I am not in full agreement. It has been observed that during the time of effective concentration, when the consciousness begins to rise above the usual level of thoughts and excludes them for a while, the breath becomes slower and more rhythmical. This is a fact which need not be contested. But the process can go much deeper, for in due time the breath will stop completely without any harm to the body of the student. Later you are given the reverse of this; for if a result of Samadhi (i.e., the deepest concentration) is the regulation and even stoppage of breath then: (a) rhythmical breathing should facilitate or (b) produce one-pointedness of the mind.

In my opinion *(a) is true* and can easily be proved, *but (b) is not quite correct* and if firmly believed can bring the danger of disappointment to the student.

I have known Hatha yogis who have perfected the domination of their breath, and by the same fact the vital energy of the body, or prana, but who were still far from any worth-while mental concentration and the ruling of thoughts by their will.

Also, there is no doubt that a suitable position of the body may contribute to more balanced thinking and so help considerably in concentration. However, the reverse of this, i.e., that some special asanas (or postures) and certain ways of breathing may create one-pointedness in your mind, or even bring you to Samadhi, as many Indians believe, is highly doubtful and experience speaks rather directly against this theory.

Many people have studied and attained great ability in performing asanas and the artificial methods of rhythmical breathing and retention of breath, and despite this have died without reaching any worth-while mind control, let alone Samadhi. In this course, the student will be given some reasonable, not cumbersome, artificial methods for breathing and sitting (i.e., pranayamas and asanas) which may be useful to him as a being still coping with physical conditions. But he should firmly remember that all of them are by no means decisive factors, as his own will power exclusively is the major one. If the student then wishes to engage in a wider and higher search, the more advanced degree of his development must be aided by the grace of a true spiritual master.

We are aware of the *power of habit* in concentration. So if you have the conviction that a certain way of sitting or breathing has contributed greatly to a well-performed exercise (see Part III), then you will probably believe that there is some connection between the two, and when next you assume that position and method of breathing, the whole mental exercise will proceed fairly well.

There is no harm in such imaginings, which will eventually disappear of themselves, when in due course you learn more about how to use pure will power to achieve your aim. Many years ago, when fighting the battle for supremacy of my mind, I found that suppression of persistent thoughts is easily achieved when the body is subjected to a sudden and unexpected shock, such as an icy-cold bath.

As a result of this discovery, I developed the habit of swimming for a few minutes in a nearby half-frozen river with its dark swollen waters flowing between snow-covered banks. There were also other things achieved by this simple practice, but stimulation of the will power was one of the most important. When you place your body in unusual and slightly dangerous conditions (for a certain element of danger always exists in such experiences), the subtle sense of separation from the body may appear, and this is the beginning of further and better things, for then you show who is boss.

There are no icy rivers where I live now, but the winter months provide a quite sufficiently low temperature in the sea water of the wide bay near my home.

Did these exercises of physical endurance bring any real ability, or were they only temporary stimulants and conditionings of outer circumstances? The student had best decide this for himself, and it should not prove difficult if he has been attentively reading this chapter.

It is not my intention to expound the innumerable techniques of yogic practices, as their name is truly legion, and every occultist is entitled to modify the existing ones and invent others. In this course you will find, in addition to the explanatory sections (which are by no means less decisive for final success than the exercises), a complete series of practical activities, some of which are apparently very similar to yogic ones. They have been arranged in order, from the elementary stages up to the most advanced and hence difficult ones. Quite a few of the latter would be very suitable for our Eastern brothers who are trying to follow the same way.

Some of the exercises, especially in the first and second series, are the same as, or parallel to, those which were known to me many years ago, when I personally found them quite adequate and reliable for the average student of concentration.

They are all based on the *training of the attention,* by fixing it on one simple object of thought, through first using the *power of visualization.* Another sort of exercise concerns sound instead of sight. Here we use the mantras or holy names, and sometimes just mere words which have nothing in common with religion. Some of these are renowned and used in many Western circles because of their simplicity and rich inner content, like "Aum" or "Om," "Hari," the famous Gayatri, names of Christ and Siva, and many others. The attention must be directed to the pronunciation of the words, which should then be said many thousands of times daily. The mind cannot be occupied with anything else but the mantra, and eventually with the counting of the number of repetitions, which is very helpful. This type of useful exercise will be found in Part III.

There is another variety of Yoga which also uses concentration, but in a different way. It is the Yoga of wisdom or Jnana Yoga. In it the meticulous exercises of the Raja Yoga and efforts to control the physical body are banned, as they are considered nonessential. The student is supposed to be sufficiently advanced to be able to use his powers of concentration for the only worthy aim—self-knowledge or self-realization. But the degree of concentration needed for such a lofty goal is infinitely greater than that required for Raja or Mantra Yoga.

Some people believe that it is impossible to practice Jnana before some degrees of Raja and Hatha Yogas have been mastered. The writer agrees with this opinion. The central idea of the Jnana Yoga is that by incessantly directing one's dynamic attention to any problem a man can arrive at the right solution.

So, by excluding everything from his consciousness as being unreal except the *bare essence of being* (rays of which are manifested in himself), man can and should reach the full achievement of his spiritual struggles. A contemporary master of the modern version of the highest Jnana gave his disciples a mighty weapon, which can break through the thick veils of ignorance in which we usually spend our lives. It is the *Vichara,* about which you will hear more in Part IV when you have already mastered the other three parts.

To resume, the Eastern methods of concentration are based firstly on the *mind's domination* and secondly on the *purification of the heart.* I speak here of the views of the eminent classical representatives of Indian Yoga like Patanjali, Sankaracharya and Sri Ramana Maharshi (the master of the Direct Path, which is not a Yoga, since it is far beyond any of them). This excludes the opinions held by the many sectarian yogis and swamis who are still in the school of Yoga and therefore are not authorities on it.

Perhaps the conception of the great Rishi Ramana Maharshi, who died only a few years ago, is more explicit. He points out that there are two ways to attainment, which he evidently supports:

Firstly, try to discover the *truth within yourself* by means of Vichara (self-inquiry); only then, when you know your true self, will you know the great Self or God and His relationship to the illusory universe.

Secondly, if you are unable to work successfully with self-inquiry, *surrender* yourself together with all your problems to the Supreme Being. If you persevere the solution will come of itself as in the first instance, and *attainment is always the same.*

Quite logically, Sri Maharshi ascribes every evil and all misery to the *primary ignorance* (i.e., sense of duality), which is the root of every trouble. Men desire and strive after many things believing that the possession of them will bring happiness. This inevitably leads to disappointment with its attendant suffering. The wise person who knows who he is and what he really needs, avoids all trouble as he is seeking for real and not temporal things.

So, from this point of view, true wisdom is the first and cardinal remedy against errors and suffering.

In this short résumé we can grasp the idea of the Eastern classical attainment and the way to it.

IX

The Western Tradition
(Heart before Mind)

As the Eastern occult schools treat concentration as a means of achieving the highest goal, so the mind takes precedence over the heart. But in the Western spiritual tradition this is reversed. The best exponents, apart from a few dissentients, fix attention first and foremost on the *moral purification* of man and his religious, devotional sense. I am not including the numerous and usually short-lived occult societies and groups, most of which were and still are occupied with aims which have practically nothing in common with the great task of transformation and purification of the human mind.

My interest has been directed to the places where men's inner work has always produced the greatest results. When I studied the lives of the first and later Christian saints of the Egyptian desert, the caves of Anatolia, the catacombs of Rome, and the monasteries of Kiev and Western Europe, I reached the firm conviction that *Western adepts knew as much as, if not more* about the value of a one-pointed mind in spiritual achievement than their Eastern brothers.

It is impossible within the framework of a book dedicated to a particular aspect of inner work, such as this, to give many examples to prove these facts, so I will mention only a few of the most interesting and striking ones.

During the third century of this era, among the hot sands and rocks of the Egyptian desert west of the Nile and also around the fertile delta of that great river were the abodes of many men of the first Christian Church—the ascetics, who were recognized as saints.

They had fled from the pagan and decadent cities which were full of immorality, in order to pursue their own way unmolested. Their practices were very different from those of the average faithful Christian. Living, as they did, so many miles from habitation, they could seldom even visit a church to hear the services because of the difficulty in walking long distances in that climate, especially for men emaciated by fasting.

Their caves and poor cells and huts were for them places of spiritual resurrection, everyday life and burial. When in India, I saw many similar caves in which, it was said, some great saint or yogi was buried, although no inscriptions revealed their names. The early Christian saints spent years in constant prayer without the complicated rituals of the sacred books, and using only a kind of mantra which they repeated all their waking hours, no matter what their bodies were engaged in at the time.

Many of them had visions which were not always pleasant and, as they said, *"did not come from God."* Sometimes these took the form of terrible temptations, often violent and of hideous appearance, which tested the saints' morale and strength of character.

In certain old chronicles, which are still extant, there is much material about the life of the well-known St. Anthony the Great, who had to face the most insidious and fierce attacks of evil. He began to lead the life of an ascetic as a young man and died well over the age of a hundred years, probably nearer 106. None of his contemporaries were able to stand the burden of aggressive evil, so frequently demonstrated in the saint's presence, and so his cave was a lonely place in the desert.

At night, visions as realistic as anything seen by day followed one after the other. Sometimes hordes of lions tried to frighten the defenseless man and on one occasion a giant whose head towered into the clouds threatened to slay him, shouting with a voice like thunder: "Where is that sinner Anthony? I will crush out his life with my feet and carry his soul into the depths of hell!" Poisonous snakes of monstrous size writhed their hideous bodies round the bare neck of the praying saint, while scorpions tried to nest in his hair. Beautiful angel-like women tried to force him to look at them in the hope of inciting him to commit a sin. But the saint knew that all these visions and visitations were only illusions arising from his own mind. He endured and left to posterity an example of the human spirit's power and strength, as have many other saints and yogis.

Among the special prayers and exorcisms which were used to combat the attacking evil forces was one that attracted my notice by its exceptional force and depth, which helped concentration more than anything I had known previously. Behind the somewhat dogmatic expression given to it by the Church, there lies hidden a deep meaning and consequent effectiveness. Moreover, this exorcism is an *impersonal* one, which greatly enhances its ethical power, since it leaves the Almighty Himself to deal with offenders and aggressors.

When slowly spoken aloud, it was believed to have the property of *immediate dissipation* of all *evil apparitions,* as well as *sinful thoughts and moods and other inner troubles.*

Before I give it, some explanation seems to be necessary. In Christian mysticism, God is considered, according to the dogmas, as omnipresent—i.e., existing in even the worst manifestation of the dark forces. But, when He is *conscious and fully active in goodness* He is considered as being in a *"dormant" state in the things we call evil.* So the word "resurrected" in the following exorcism has a very deep meaning. Perhaps it would be better to use the term "awakened," but who are we to change the tradition of almost eighteen hundred years?

> May God be resurrected and His foes vanish.
> As wax melts before fire, as smoke is dispersed by the
>   wind,
> So may all who hate the Lord flee from His sight,
> And the just rejoice!

This is a literal translation from the old Greek, because in such texts the exactness seems to be more important than the smooth outer form of the words. It is still occasionally used in the Greek Orthodox Church, and great powers are ascribed to this old verse as a *guard against the evil will, inner troubles, temptations and mental disturbances.*

Of course, effective use of the words implies strong concentration, and this is just the *motive force* which acts. But our will may also be strongly stimulated by other suitable outer means, thus enabling us to reach a level of concentration we never before knew.

If used with faith and strength, the above exorcism may be of value to students who experience serious difficulty in creating the "astral or odic armor" (see last paragraphs of Chapter XVIII). I would also like to quote another mantra in the form of a short prayer which is used in both Western and Eastern Christian churches:

> God the Holy, Holy and Mighty, Holy and Immortal—be
>   gracious unto me!

This was and is still used in some monasteries and is repeated thousands of times daily, often with the name of Christ added.

If you read the meditations and instructions of St. Ignatius Loyola written by him for the members of the order which he founded, it is certain that, providing you are acquainted with them, you will immediately think of Raja and Bhakti Yogas.

The building up of mental pictures of tremendous reality by concentration and the creation (by the same means) of currents of emotion directed into certain channels of consciousness, all of which are described before the actual exercises, will show you whether the Eastern Yogas have any monopoly in their ideas, methods and results.

The methods of "mental travel" used in some occult manuals as a means for one-pointedness have their equivalents, although perhaps more pronounced, in the famous Loyola exercises.

In his life and wisdom, the East Russian saint, Seraphim of Sarov, was one of the greatest and most interesting. He taught an almost direct combination of Raja and Mantra Yoga to his pupil-monks. He advised them to repeat the already mentioned short prayer (the second quoted above) at first one thousand times daily, increasing to two thousand, and then later to three and more until seven thousand was reached. At the same time he advised the use of a morning and evening exercise for trying to retain the breath for fairly long periods while incessantly repeating the same prayer inwardly. When demonstrating this, Seraphim said: "You will feel a wonderful warmth in your heart, and the repetition will soon become automatic and easy." Many Hindu swamis firmly believe that they may reach Samadhi by practicing the rhythmical retention of breath for as long as they can. Who then actually possesses the "copyright" for such methods?

While I was in India I heard of some yogis and even yoginis who were sealed up alive in caves on the slopes of a holy mountain, and who received only a little food through a small window or hole in a wall.

In 1918 when I was occasionally in Kiev, the ancient capital of the Ukraine, I used to visit the famous old monastery of Petchersk, built about seven hundred years ago, whose subterranean galleries went deep under the River Dnieper. On both sides of the passages were single cells, some with only a little square hole in place of a door. It was said that at one time these cells used to house great ascetics, who spent many years in darkness and solitude praying both day and night. One of the monks told me that in such cases the only means of knowing whether or not the hermit was still alive was by the untouched food left for him in the window-like hole.

I was shown some of their bodies, taken from the cells many years after their deaths. They lay in open coffins in the usual modest black clothes of monks, with thin parchment-like faces and wax-yellow hands crossed on their breasts. But there were *no signs of decomposition* and no smell of decay. "How did they spend their long lives?" I asked the prior. "Only repeating the holy name of Christ" was the answer. An unrivaled example of a perfect combination of Mantra and Bhakti Yogas.

I think that many famous Indian yogis of the past would have liked to have known their advanced Western brethren.

In the earliest as well as the more recent chronicles of the lives of the saints, we find a record of many mysterious happenings which we call miracles. I am referring to the cures and other superphysical activities of those few "friends of God," as Paul Sédir so beautifully styled them. There is no room here nor purpose in enumerating many of them, so I shall limit the examples to one which is the most striking because of its superb simplicity, authenticity and modesty, so typical of the Christian saints of the highest order. The scientific elimination of the mortal ego personality in man, as taught by the great Rishi Ramana, also shines here, but in a different form.

When St. Seraphim of Sarov was middle-aged, the fame of his cures and other miraculous activities in restoring the inner human balance became widely known in the district surrounding the saint's hut.

The then governor was hopelessly bedridden with paralyzed limbs and at the time, according to the doctors, death was only a few weeks distant. His wife desperately tried the last hope by taking her husband to St. Seraphim. The following account of that strange visit is taken from the still preserved official records.

When the coach carrying the dying nobleman was still some two or three hours' riding distance away, St. Seraphim said to his disciples: "General K. is coming to seek for God's Grace. Sweep the clearing round the hut [it was set in the forest] and prepare a place for His Excellency to sit." The monks placed the only available chair outside the saint's humble dwelling. When the coach arrived the servants brought the helpless man before St. Seraphim and placed him in the waiting chair.

"How do you do, Your Excellency!" said the smiling saint. The patient who could only speak with great difficulty murmured: "I am dying, my Father. I can no longer move. Have pity on me." "Who told you such things," laughingly said Seraphim. "I think you will be better if you come for a walk, for the air in this forest of ours is very good."

"Why do you mock me, Father? You see that I am unable to move even one step," sadly replied the Governor. "All right, all right, but we shall try it in God's name." And so saying, the saint took the sick man's hand in his own meager palm and gently raised the inert body from its seat. "Now walk with me, do not fear for I am holding you," said Seraphim.

And the old man, who weighed about fifteen stone, began to walk around the clearing beside the saint, with every step becoming firmer. "I can walk! I can walk!" he cried, as if scarcely able to credit the miracle. "Yes, and you walk very well, Excellency. Go on! Go on! A little more practice will do you good." "I can even run, can't I?" "Yes, it is God's will that you will be all right now," remarked the smiling Seraphim.

Then the saint took the cured man into his hut for a few minutes as if for a chat; but when they reappeared, those present saw a peculiar, inspired expression on the formerly pain-marked face of the Governor. All were silent.

The official took leave of his benefactor, prostrating on the earth before the serene Seraphim. But the saint was by no means pleased with the gesture and he quickly lifted the Governor saying to him: "What are you doing, Excellency? I am only God's servant, a man like yourself. It is God who should be praised and worshiped, not His servants."

Seraphim, who was approximately the same age as the Governor, outlived him by only a year or two. When the death of his pupil was reported to him, he remarked: "Now the time is also coming for Seraphim. I hope we shall meet again where no sickness or sadness exists any more."

Through the following centuries, many miracles have occurred at the graveside of the saint.

In the lives of the Eastern saints and yogis there have not been many similar examples of this kind of service and help given to those around them. Probably because many of them were so indifferent toward things physical.

From the foregoing we can see that the laws governing inner human strength are as well known and applied in the West as in the East. Only, in the Western countries the heart aspect predominates, and the mind's subordination follows later. This means that it is recognized—not without good reason—that *first* must come the *purification and strengthening* of the seat of human emotions, which often creates so many difficulties for aspirants to spirituality. The seat of our moral law must first be balanced, and then order comes to dwell in the pure heart. It is then that the development of the mind's powers cannot be dangerous, either for their owners or for their surroundings.

The West still remembers with caution the misuse of powers of concentration by immoral men (black magicians). In the East even renowned authors like Patanjali and Sankaracharya seem to be less concerned about the question. They claim that any psychic powers worth mentioning are too hard to develop without an adequate moral standard having been reached beforehand. One may or may not agree with this idea, for in the past there has been a great deal known about the use of the fruits of concentration for illegal purposes and this is still the case.

In this realm, as everywhere, there exists a safety valve which controls the activities and numbers of those eager to possess psychical powers, which in India are called "siddhis." It is—endurance.

Human nature is so arranged that for petty or doubtful aspirations in inner training one usually lacks the necessary stamina for the effort. Therefore, evil in occultism is always restricted *to a certain degree* by the weakness and lack of pure aims on the part of the prospective black magician.

However, as such a person is necessarily a materialist, since all lower aims invariably have a body as their base, then sickness or death of that body may put an end to the mischievous career, leaving the man with a formidable account to settle for his misdeeds. There is only one form of payment for such a debt. Its name is suffering, no matter whether in this or other worlds.

In my youth I read a terrible book, a unique and rare volume from an edition of only a few copies, written by the once well-known occultist—Stanislas de Guaita of Paris. In this large work was explained how to perform various occult practices complete with all the techniques. Among them was a kind of necromancy as well as the exteriorization of the astral body of a living person and its projection, with the intention of influencing others for the operator's own purposes, without any fear of judicial retribution. The law still does not officially recognize most occult phenomena and activities, according them merely the status of superstition. In spite of this the danger exists.

Recipes containing rare but procurable drugs were given

which could—and should, as the author advised—produce the most deplorable effects, including death, *if misused or wrongly applied.* Fortunately, even for such malicious deeds a considerable degree of the same *ability of concentration is always needed.* And not everyone is able or willing to develop the dangerous ability, so that more bungling than real magic is the outcome.

While the black magicians of the West put themselves in opposition to good (as a manifestation of God) and to religion, in the East there seems to have been a less obvious demarcation between the two poles of good and evil. This does not apply to the greatest spirits of the East, such as the ancient and modern rishis, who are beyond all reproach and blame.

It may be useful for you to know something more definite about siddhis, which are so much discussed in occult circles.

As a definition, we may assume that siddhis, also called occult powers or psychical forces, consist of *everything* which cannot be practically or theoretically explained by known physical laws, or laws as yet unknown but in the course of discovery.

One of their peculiarities is that they transcend physical laws and the results of their application cannot be explained by those laws. Telepathy, hypnotism, thought reading, miracle cures, transportation of solid objects without any physical means, apparent creation of such objects from nothing (or so it seems to our five senses), use of languages never heard before, second sight or ability to foresee past or future events—all of these and many other things could be termed psychical powers.

Perhaps in no other subdivision of human knowledge does there reign such disorder or lack of a system, as in occult problems. Therefore, when the student comes into touch with siddhis, he sometimes feels as if he were in a dense forest of mixed and unexplained facts.

To begin with, we will define two aspects of siddhis—involuntary and voluntary. The first one is the most commonly known. Many of us have had presentiments of events far ahead in time, which were later fulfilled; had "intuitional" knowledge of another person's thoughts, and experienced strange dreams which later proved to be a hint to one's most intimate inner world. Cases have been known where the presence of certain people has had an unquestionable influence on the health or well-being of others. In all such instances the phenomena cannot be produced at will: they are only happenings, chances and nothing more. We may experience them only once in our lives or many times; but always *we are not in control of them.* Of course, men try to find one or another explanation, according to their mentality and inclinations. But they can only guess and not arrive at any definite findings on the causes of the phenomena. Some people have seen an apparition of a distant friend or relative and then later received news of the death or of a peculiar accident affecting that person, and even if *they had wished* to know, they could not *otherwise* have learned anything about the person apart from letters or communications from others.

By the foregoing remarks I want to underline the involuntary character of most psychic occurrences. I have known people who possessed an involuntary ability to cure certain diseases by the use of touch or prayer. If such people are honest with themselves, they must freely acknowledge their ignorance about the causes and proceedings which create such phenomena. At the same time, some of them invent different theories which apparently support their guesses. But they cannot *always* produce their abilities at will, and so they say that "some conditions are favorable—or unfavorable." Then, because they have nothing definite to work with, they never try to possess the occult powers by the practice of exercises in order to develop them.

As such types of siddhis are exempt from any logical or scientific examination we may leave them alone and pass on to another variety, i.e., to the *siddhis acquired by definite and direct efforts,* such as those practiced by different occult schools in both East and West. Lower kinds of Indian Yoga are also occupied with the same purpose. Men who try to acquire occult powers always do it in order to influence others or even themselves. Listen to what the Master Sri Maharshi has to say of such people:

"All siddhis need two conditions: the *person* who exercises them and the *others* who may see them; therefore, there is duality and not unity. As duality is only an illusion, so all such siddhis invariably belong to the realm of illusion. They are, indeed, only temporary and do not exist forever. Whatever does not possess the attribute of permanence is only illusory and therefore not worth striving to obtain."

The rishi pointed out the true aim of life when he said: "The spiritual power of self-realization is infinitely greater than all the siddhis put together.

". . . Do not think too much of psychical phenomena and such things. Their number is legion; clairvoyance, clairaudience and such things are not worth having, when so much far greater illumination and peace of mind are possible without them than with them. The master takes on these powers as a form of self-sacrifice! The master becomes only the instrument of God, and when his mouth opens it speaks God's words without effort or forethought; and when he raises a hand, God flows again through that, to work a miracle.

"The idea that a master is simply one who has attained power over the various occult senses by long practice and prayer or anything of the kind, is absolutely false. No true master ever cared a rap for occult powers, for he has no need of them in his daily life.

"Do not fix your attention on all these changing things of

life, death and phenomena. Do not think even of the actual act of seeing or perceiving them, but only of *that* which sees all these things—*that which is responsible* for it all [i.e., the unique self]."

Nevertheless, those who are strong and persistent enough to achieve concentration often notice that these siddhis actually begin to manifest in them.

As Sri Maharshi said: "The results of concentration (Vichara) will be seen *in all sorts of unconscious* clairvoyance, in peace of mind, in power to deal with troubles, in power all around, yet always *unconscious* power."

The persons who obtain these *unconscious* powers never feel that "they are the ones using the siddhis." And why? Simply because they do not believe in the old myth of their ego personality. Therefore, the thought that such and such an individual who bears their name, possesses the siddhis, cannot flourish in their consciousness. If this were not a fact, then realization would still be a very distant thing for such men, because they would not as yet have transcended the illusion of the separate perishable being.

To recapitulate we can say that:

1. The uncontrollable and accidental phenomena exhibited by some people, who are not engaged in any particular spiritual search, are not worthy of our attention.

2. The striving after these occult powers as an aim is wrong and does not take us closer to the spiritual realization of being. There is always a great danger of creating a *powerful ego* which could be substituted (in the eyes of such a mistaken person) for the true aim of the perennial realization—the immortal Truth.

3. There is a possibility for a person who enters on the path of realization to have some occult senses and powers appear, but without any effort or striving on his part. He would never exhibit such powers before anyone, for he ignores them, con-

sidering them unworthy of mention. In the *Voice of the Silence* by Madame H. P. Blavatsky, it is said of a disciple approaching close to the final liberation: "Acquiring the siddhis in the course of his previous path, he will again consciously renounce all of them."

4. There exists a mysterious spiritual siddhi or power which only a perfect master can possess. It is the ability, unaided by any special words or deeds, to help and promote the evolution of his disciple's consciousness. It is actually unexplainable; but I believe it to be something like an invisible radiation which can reach to the deepest recesses of the disciple's soul. Then, if the man is able to tune this consciousness to the vibrations of the master's spirit, he *knows* many things which remain hidden from others. But he does not know the way in which the light reaches him, and is indifferent to the cause of it. He is quite satisfied with the mere *fact itself,* and nothing else is of any interest.

For a discriminating man there is no absolute cure for disease in any Yoga, medical science, so-called spiritual healing, etc., of which, nowadays, we hear so much and read in numerous advertisements. Western occultism as well as Eastern Yoga often claim their methods to be all-curing or disease preventives. But when the authors fall ill, which sooner or later usually happens to them as with most people, they nearly always hurry to make full use of official medical science by taking drugs, injections and inoculations. I know of many such examples.

They also die much about the same age as average men despite their assertions (in books) that by following their methods, men may enjoy perfect health and live to an almost incredible age. But everything is limited in this physical world. Doctors cannot always help, but at least *they are honest enough to admit the fact.*

Spiritual healers and others probably effect far less a percentage of cures than do doctors, but by comparison, they publicize their successful cases far too much. Even Christ did not cure all the sick and disabled when He walked amongst us in Palestine.

Where then lies help? In the clear understanding that: *A man who according to his karma has to be cured of his affliction* will surely find the right doctor, a suitable "spiritual healer," or a yogic book to follow, no matter what it may be; *but if it is not meant to be,* i.e., if the man cannot avoid his disease or death, *help will not be forthcoming from any source.*

Lourdes, famous for its many miracle cures, does not restore the health of all the thousands seeking relief, but only of an infinitesimal number of the persons who pray in the miraculous grotto. If you have understood all this, you will be reasonable about the needs of your physical shell, and will never madly pursue different systems and methods of occult healing.

When stricken by disease, the great saints do not usually seek a cure, for they have practical *knowledge* of the source of suffering and infirmity and their meaning.

So it would be a mistake for an average man to ascribe an infallible effectiveness to any medical or occult treatment, as all such things are only relatively helpful. Whoever claims the opposite is deceiving himself, or as more often happens—others.

From our point of view, physical and other afflictions are only necessary lessons, unavoidable until one has learned them in full. There does, however, exist in the higher degrees of occult (rather than spiritual) wisdom a means which can apparently dispose of even incurable diseases. It is when one deliberately learns in advance the lesson which is to cause misery. Then it becomes unnecessary, just as it would be pointless to send a graduate back to an elementary school, for he has nothing to learn from it.

This is that mysterious and usually much misunderstood "burning up of past karma" by certain actions and inner work. It is possible, but only in very rare cases, as it calls for an exceptional intelligence and knowledge of laws which are inaccessible to the majority of us.

I know of an example where a man was stricken with a disease, incurable from the medical point of view, but who was healed without any outer help or attempt to obtain it. When asked to explain the incredible fact, he answered simply: "I only accepted the coming test with all its consequences, fully known to me, without trying to avoid anything which might happen. Then perhaps, because it was no longer necessary, there was no further reason for the disease to appear."

And the statement made nearly two thousand years ago came to my mind:

"Not even a hair dares to fall from your head without My Father's will. . . ."

To realize this means to reach the inner peace.

X

Obstacles and Aids

The chief obstacle to concentration is the uncontrolled emotional nature of the average untrained man. In the Eastern tradition there is a handy word for these uncontrolled elements —"vasanas," or innate mental and astral tendencies. Vasanas can be both good and evil, and *all of them are obstacles* to the higher degrees of concentration. Therefore, for this study, *both kinds are unwanted,* and they should at least be controlled.

In other words, we should be able to choose from among these vibrations just what we actually need for our everyday life and definitely refuse to occupy ourselves with them when we have better work to do. What results can I expect from my exercises if I am unable, at the desired moment, to stop my anger or greed against someone near me and consequently think ceaselessly about him? Or if I am occupied with lustful thoughts and cannot break the unclean chain?

I may be so unreasonably attached to my family that, for example, from my egotistical point of view, I imagine that I have to be continually anxious about its welfare, forgetting that every human being has his own destiny and karma, which no one can influence beyond the narrow limits of his activities. The result is that I am *unable to stop the unnecessary and per-*

sistent thoughts in order to begin work on my fifteen minutes of exercises. Those deliberations about the clothes I have to buy for my son tomorrow, or about a birthday gift for my wife, etc., can claim plenty of my time apart from these few minutes.

The vasanas, then, are the first *serious obstacle* which must be pitilessly destroyed if we want to raise our inner status by the study of concentration.

A weak state of physical health can also be a serious hurdle for beginners. Usually such people tend to identify themselves with their bodies, and being physically defective, they feel the same in their thoughts and emotions, i.e., in the astral and mental planes. Without some inner strength no study is possible. Therefore such people would do better if they abandoned their ambitions to become stronger *in this way,* because it is not appropriate for them. A life of *surrender to the Highest* is as effective as that of the Direct Path and much more suited to them.

Another obstacle is "instinctive materialism" on the part of the prospective student. At the present time there are still many individuals who are unable to believe or to feel something which they cannot touch or see. These studies are also not for them, because without a sense of subtle things, the result will be void.

To be in the power of superstition is a very serious hindrance, barring us from any success. This vice is nothing less than a kind of slavery of our mind, compelled to think in a faulty way. Fanaticism also often comes to the aid of its unholy brother—superstition.

Intolerance belongs to the same unpleasant family of handicaps. Imagine a fanatical and intolerant sectarian or religious bigot reading these chapters. How much material to condemn he would find in them! And by so doing, such people would lose any trust they might have had in the matters discussed, plus developing an unreasonable contempt for the writer. How could they then perform the exercises in this book?

Still another barrier for many people which closes the door to success is the mania or passion for reading too many books, because of their inability to make a definite choice. Getting one on a theme which interests them, they invariably soon seek something "new," and as soon as that has been read, they again start their interminable searching. Their lives pass without being properly and reasonably used.

Such men forget that books are much more numerous than the weeks and months they have yet to live through. So what is the good of having read even half of them and dying before making any use of the things which men know only mentally?

After all, books are usually for us only crystallized stores of borrowed thoughts created by other men, and not always of use to us, since in all fields of literature they so frequently offer only fiction or near-fiction, which can hardly help an earnest seeker.

Although the mind is only a secondary power in man, compared with the higher wisdom consciousness known in Samadhi, which is devoid of thoughts, faults in the structure of that mind are almost an absolute barrier impossible to overcome in any study, and especially in the present one. Inadequate comprehension is the same as insufficient knowledge of a foreign alphabet for someone who wants to read in that particular language.

It may happen that it is not merely an unquenchable thirst for reading which drives a man from one author to another, but the fact that he is not satisfied with any so far encountered. In such a case there is nothing more to say then: "Seek and ye shall find."

Addicts of drunkenness or other habit-forming vices cannot possibly hope to be students of concentration for the simple reason that their real *will power is too close to zero.* If they cannot stop their bad habits, which they know perfectly well are harmful for them, where then would they find enough *inner strength* to overcome their mental apathy and laziness?

Excessive nervousness is a sickness which may easily affect the will power of a man. It should be successfully treated before an effective study can be undertaken. The study of concentration itself is *not a remedy for all our faults*. On the other hand, an average man, not affected by any of the above-mentioned blemishes of character or body, will undoubtedly enjoy a fair reward from an earnestly undertaken study of the subject.

Now, what may be most helpful for the student?

In contemporary occult and psychological literature we find an excess of "aids" in all directions. Everyone speaks only about the things which were apparently very helpful to him and everyone is endlessly seeking for help and still more help. It is wrong of course. If people decided to walk only with the aid of sticks or crutches, their limbs would soon become weak and useless. This faulty attitude of the present day is based on the subconscious belief that something from outside may be added to pull us as a mother cat pulls her kitten by its neck. It is basically a *lack of faith* in man's own inner strength and value. Be careful, and do not succumb to this malady.

Anyway, speaking practically, the lack of all these vices and imperfections is the best help a man can have, and the presence of virtues is the most favorable of conditions. But one thing is of overwhelming value for the prospective student: a capacity for quiet, cold and clear thinking and judgment about life in general. Next in importance is sincere interest in possessing the abilities given by concentration.

Sometimes the prospective student knows why he wants to participate in such a course. But it may also happen that he does not, but simply feels a strong urge to do so. This is also quite a good condition, as there is every likelihood that the highest principle in man is driving him on, without expressing itself through the mind. Another genuine help is to read inspiring books written by men who themselves have passed through many difficulties in their lives, but who have finally experienced the Truth and landed safely on the shore whose blessed name is attainment.

It would be an exceptional privilege in this life to encounter the teachings and authentic words of a true spiritual master. If well understood, the light of such a revelation might easily enlighten the darkest corners of our still unknown and undiscovered inner being.

I will deliberately refrain from describing the great benefits to a student should this supreme opportunity occur—i.e., the encountering of a master in his physical form. Such an event could make all studies, including this one, unnecessary and obsolete. I shall return to this question in Chapter XXII.

But actually, at the present time, there is little likelihood of seeing a true master alive on this earth, for one departed only a few years ago, and they do not come too often. The waiting for their advent may exceed many lives and thousands of years.

XI

Inner Attitude—the Key to Attainment

The title of this chapter is a positive one. In the invisible world where our *feelings and thoughts* function, as well as the spirit of the *inner unchangeable essence,* "attitude" is dual, and often even composed of all three of these factors. Our attitude is very much akin to what we really are. We obviously still do not possess self-knowledge for otherwise we would need no training in concentration. But we are able to perceive, even to change, our attitude toward the outer and inner things encountered in life.

And therein lies the greatest chance of success.

The true key to every achievement lies in the ability to look deeply into things, their sequence and their relation to ourselves. The summit of right attitude was stressed many times by those earlier spiritual brothers of present-day men. The Christ called it the Perfect Truth, and ascribed to it all possible powers. "If you have faith as a grain of mustard seed, you shall say to this mountain: Remove from hence hither, and it shall remove . . ."

Such a faith cannot be expected or required of beginners, but at least they should have a *positive attitude* toward this work, which is solely in the interest of the student himself. I am not suggesting that there should be "blind faith" in my statements, but only an honest investigation, deliberation and decision about them.

If you lack a positive attitude, even after your mental efforts to acquire one, then it may be a sign that this is not your path. No dogmatic assertion is intended that the way given in this book is the only one—or even the shortest or easiest leading to the goal. Not at all! This also will be explained, when you finish your training, at the end of Chapter XXI.

But it is *one of the safest paths,* which cannot be dangerous, and always contributes some inner progress, even if you are unable to perform all the advance series of exercises.

When just about thirty years ago I began my first practical course in concentration in a little book of the same title, I had almost unlimited confidence that I would succeed in performing all the exercises, and thereby obtain some wonderful results. As it happened, I had no definite idea what these would be, for the booklet spoke little about the ultimate target of the study.

As long as I worked at my exercises, everything seemed to be all right; but when chapters on concentration were followed by others expounding meditation, confusion entered, and I saw only a dead end confronting me. The cause of this is now quite clear. There was too wide a gap between the elementary exercises—which could not confer any special abilities on me at that stage—and the abstract and ready-made ideas, borrowed from what was to me at the time an alien philosophy.

Today I have lost my enthusiasm for that book, as I cannot see any real aim in it. Then came another one, much more serious and advanced. The exercises were very difficult; but they *could* give the earnest student new abilities, and there was quite a clear explanation of the means to the final goal.

It is true that the study cost me years of strenuous work, as a result of which I have included among the advanced series in this volume some modified exercises taken from Dr. Brand-ler-Pracht's manual.

Just as the *attitude* of the student is of *first importance* to success, so the duty of the author is to help his readers, without allowing any good approach to be spoiled by his lack of personal experience. Hence one of the safeguards is suitable preparation and explanation of the matter before passing to the exercises. That is why less than one-third of the chapters in this book have been devoted to the purely technical side of things.

XII

What Is the Mind?

This question is far from easy to answer properly. But as we operate with the power of mind (and you should certainly have no doubts that it is a kind of power), we are entitled to know how to define it, according to its actual functions.

It would be useless to write extended definitions, because for everyday use you need something concise. What I now quote comes from the late Rishi Ramana, the modern authority on the subject, and I could not find anything better than the sage's statement:

Mind is only a bundle of thoughts: stop thinking and show me, then, where is the mind?

This is a perfect philosophical equation, which contains the full practical solution in itself. Let us analyze the first part of it, which indicates that the power of the mind manifests itself only in the thinking process. That is already a partial elimination of the unknown "X," for I can think, thereby I can experience action, the very property of "X."

The next part is clearer still. The mind is nothing more than a collection, *the sum total of thoughts*. Of course, this statement also contains the unconditional solution which refers to

76

all three subdivisions of time. Hence the mind is: the thoughts which have already been had; the thoughts now in our minds; and the thoughts which will come into our consciousness in the future, or of those who will live on after our departure.

The eternal "bundle of thoughts," as the sage tells us, remains. He wished to eliminate any possibility of doubt in us. This makes the last part of the equation devoid of all compromise: "If you do not believe, then stop your thinking and try to find the mind."

Experience will show that what remains is unlike that "mind." This brings another important sequence to light: the mind does not have an independent existence, unaffected by the attitude of beings able to think. Again a revelation! If all this is so, then there cannot be any doubt that *man is able to conquer the mind* and to direct it according to his own will. The mind is a finite and hence limited quantity, therefore it can be controlled.

We will attempt to gain this control in the chapters that follow. In essence, mind is rather like a neutral sort of energy, not evil, not good. Simply, I would like to state that mind likes to vibrate, no matter whether these vibrations (i.e., thoughts) are considered by beings like ourselves to be either good or bad.

Here vasanas enter the picture. Predisposition is the filter which allows certain kinds of vibrations endowed with these vasanas to enter the brain's consciousness—while at the same time it drives other kinds of thoughts and feelings from the doorway of our consciousness.

Therefore, a saint would not be impressed by the dirty astral or mental atmosphere of a hotel bar or cabaret, while a man who is a prey to his vasanas would be fully influenced and would expand them by the work of his imagination and emotions. In this way a ripe soul will immediately and intuitively discover the greatness of a saint or a master of wisdom, whereas an unripe person might easily pass them by without any visible reaction, as in a dream.

What then is the explanation of the famous verse of the *Viveka-Chudamani:* "Therefore the mind is the cause of the bondage of this individual and also of his liberation. The mind when stained by passion is the cause of bondage, and of liberation when pure, devoid of passion and ignorance."

From the Maharshi's "equation" of mind we can conclude that man *IS in a position to separate himself from his mind,* from that mere "bundle of thoughts." Moreover, by this fact itself, he can select his own kind of thoughts. Now apply this finding to Sankaracharya's aphorism, and you may see that both bondage and liberation are nowhere save within you.

Which of them do you accept and invite, and which do you reject and repel? That is what no one else can know or do for you except yourself, just as *no one* can take medicine in order that *you* may be cured. *Sapienti sat,* dear reader.

Until comparatively recently, essential knowledge of the mind was farthest advanced in the East, especially in Indian philosophical works of the past. The attitude of the true Indian masters to this power is clear and concise, as you can perhaps see for yourself from the analysis of the Rishi Ramana's statements on the subject.

The West still lags behind, at least in its official knowledge, which only operates with theories and guesses. It is more interested in peculiar functions of, and phenomena (often pathological) produced by, the human mind than in its very essence. That is only natural! Mind cannot discover the mind!

Something superior must supplant it before the seeker can be enlightened. Western psychological science with all its innumerable conceptions really has little experimental and experiential knowledge about the constitution of the human mind. Nowadays, new currents of thought entering Western psychology are coming from the old Hindu Advaitic philosophy and these are vividly discussed and dissected in European scientific circles. But for the purpose of this study we need little more than has already been told. The true experimental knowledge will be yours as a result of the duly performed exercises of Part III.

That "something superior" is the power which enables us *to know* and to act rightly *without thinking,* i.e., without the mind's active participation.

Now let us analyze another aspect of the mind's functions. Human beings are often confronted with, and are usually interested in, the manifestations of that power (mind) which directly affect them. This is quite understandable, since the physical tool or "filter" through which we are able to establish a contact with the acting mind is our brain, just as the nervous system is the conductor of feelings or astral activities.

In mentally deficient individuals, scientists have discovered different abnormalities present in the structure of their brains. On occasions surgery is used in an attempt to rectify the deficiencies of these ailing organs. Malignant tumors can also affect a man's mental abilities, as does any damage inflicted on certain important centers in the brain. There have been cases where formerly brilliant and highly intelligent men have lost their powers because of physical changes in their brains, due to disease or loss of a portion of their gray matter, following accidents or unsuccessful operations.

In some such unfortunate cases, the persons concerned have even become hopeless idiots, lacking every trace of their former intelligence and culture. These are facts, and in them we can find another support for the assertion that, in the ultimate sense, the mental and astral planes are still material (although subtle) and dependent on physical matter for their manifestation.

Therefore a man's consciousness, provided he is average, does not yet possess any supermental (i.e., spiritual) awareness in this life, which is limited to the mind-brain's activities.

Speaking practically, what happens when not only a part but the whole of the brain is destroyed, as inevitably occurs with death? You may answer the question for yourself!

Persons who have temporarily lost the link between their astral counterpart and physical body because of anaesthetics (as in operations) often report that their conscious existence was then limited to dreaming and sometimes even to a full dimming of all awareness. This link is also permanently severed at death.

It is worth thinking deeply about these facts, instead of accepting the innumerable occult theories which cannot be tested personally.

By subduing both elements (i.e., astral and mental) while still living, we logically open the gate to a new life, which makes us independent of the perishable shells we now use.

But this wisdom must invariably be obtained *here and now,* for it is evident from the foregoing that death cannot bring us any additional knowledge, which has had no prior existence.

That is why all our advanced brethren, whom we call saints and sages, were and are so anxious *to get that wisdom now,* and to teach us *to do the same,* as the only real safeguard against the darkness of death.

XIII

Different Aspects of Consciousness

While writing these pages, I am in the so-called "waking state of consciousness," or Jagrat in Hindu terminology. In it I am in contact with the outer world by means of my five senses. I see, hear, taste, smell and touch. If one of them fails, my perception of events and activities in the world becomes the poorer by the subtraction of the affected sense.

We can presume that a human being who has lost all the five senses becomes insensible to the outer world.

Therefore, the physical senses and the world are interdependent. If the latter does not impress itself on our consciousness in any way, it no longer exists as an experience for our consciousness. The *memory of former impressions* still contained in the brain does not affect this statement; for *imagination* belonging to the past, present or future *is not experience*. It is more akin to the dream world, which cannot be taken into consideration. All that we know about the waking state is reflected in our relative consciousness, and it is just that factor which makes decisions about the form of the world and its manifestations.

If we were limited to this aspect of consciousness and no other, then we could speak about the unity of the world's manifestation, and consequently try to prove the reality of outward things on the ground of their uniformity, i.e., by the only known and conceivable state of consciousness.

In Jagrat I move, speak, feel, act, think and so on as others do. It seems to be perfectly simple and logical, and it would be if there were no other states in which we could equally live and act. One of them is fairly well known to us, we believe. It is the state of dream during sleep, in which we still have the idea of "I" and "Non-I," or "I" and all the "other things" that constitute the physical world. But what we experience in dreams, where the former world of Jagrat has disappeared and cannot be found, is very different from what we experience in the waking state. Things become possible which are obviously impossible when we are awake, and activities of the waking state have little effect on the dream state—although to a certain extent there is a kind of interdependence between the two states. In Indian terminology the dream state is called Swapna.

One cold night I had a horrible dream in which I was trapped by a mountain landslide with great masses of earth pressing on my chest and suffocating me. The nightmare was so real that I awoke, and immediately discovered the cause of it: my pet cat had decided that it would be much warmer for her if she slipped under the blankets, curled up on my chest and put her paws round my neck.

Subsequently, when at night I had to accept this sort of co-operation against the cold, the nightmare did not recur, probably because the subconscious mind working in the state of dream was instructed by its waking brother that there was no danger in my cat's habits.

Sometimes unusual odors in our rooms can produce a particular kind of dream. On occasions when I have left sticks of Indian incense burning in my bedroom, I have often dreamed of being in a temple and watching puja (a kind of Hindu mass), and other incidents from my life in the East have also returned in my dreams.

Leaving our feet uncovered during cold weather will often cause us to dream of standing in water or on ice. There are many other tricks known to psychologists, but this is not the place to quote them. It should be enough to know that a mutual dependence between our physical state and the resultant dreams does exist. This is not meant to imply that *all dreams* are necessarily the direct results of the physical conditions of the sleeping form at the time of dreaming. Indeed, the majority of dreams do not belong to this category at all. But what we have to realize is that in the sleeping state we do not use our five physical senses, yet a lot of impressions still enter our consciousness while the senses are "switched off."

The next state of consciousness or awareness—if it is possible to speak of any awareness in it—is that mysterious state of dreamless sleep, or Sushupti in Indian terms, which is totally dissimilar to the two states known to us, waking and dreaming.

Usually, we have no remembrance of any kind of our experiences in Sushupti. It remains an apparently insoluble enigma.

Even so, we continued to exist during that gap in our memory. We simply cannot accept that we ceased to be.

The enlightening of the dark corners of our consciousness is actually possible through the use of our *expanded abilities,* which can be gained only by the *practice of concentration,* leading us in the end to a life without sensation or thought. Only then can we penetrate and illuminate what is still darkness for us.

As an average man, untrained in concentration, cannot lift himself beyond his thoughts and feelings (the mental and astral planes), so he cannot willfully raise himself into the rarefied atmosphere of Sushupti, until he takes some appropriate steps in that direction. Part III gives the necessary instructions in this matter. When you study Chapters XIX and XX, remember this, so that the things mentioned here may be recalled before the tribunal of your consciousness, then widened by the exercises of that part of the course.

Now, what is the aim of concentration seen from the above point of view? It is to enable you to pass *consciously* from the three lower states (i.e., waking, dream and dreamless sleep) into the *fourth,* which is above and beyond the others. This fourth state (Turiya) is the final one, the peak and the goal. Do not be worried by the different theories of some occult societies, which like to multiply the higher states ad infinitum, some even speaking of forty-nine different planes, which *only exist in the imagination of their authors.*

To each type of thought they often ascribe a whole "new plane of existence," though they themselves have not even had conscious experience of Sushupti, let alone Turiya. The more you really know, the more you admire the *superb simplicity of things* as seen with the eye of wisdom, in place of differences and multiplicity.

From the Turiya, as from a high mountain, one sees through the three lower states, at the same time being independent of them. This state cannot be reached without stilling the senses and the mind, and this is what the student must fully realize. If he does not, but still entertains any hope that he may "slip in through a side entrance," *he is deceiving himself,* and consequently will have to pay for it. The currency for payment of our mistakes is only one. Its name is suffering!

Everything mentioned in this chapter affects all "normal" cases, which means that we have to work in order to obtain abilities which we do not as yet possess and which we recognize to be very necessary. So, just like a school curriculum, this course has been planned, written and explained.

From the last chapters we will learn something of the circumstances under which one can immediately get the needed abilities without passing through the normal process of evolutive learning. However, these cases are so rare and unpredictable that to count on them or place any hope in them would be as unreasonable as hoping to avoid earning a living in the usual way by winning a big lottery prize or making some other gambling coup.

The fourth state of consciousness or Turiya is, from the point of view of the average man, the superconsciousness. But for those who have attained it and managed to live in it, Turiya —or in other words, the Sahaja Nirvikalpa Samadhi (perennial formless superconsciousness or ecstasy)—is a normal everyday experience, and all other lower states are for them utterly unreal, narrow and limited. Such men can never take the viewpoint of Jagrat or Sushupti as the basis of their experience.

Now, knowing something about the different states of consciousness in man, the student will gain another step toward the understanding of the aims and methods of concentration. This can only be welcomed, for the greater our grasp of the object of this study, the less likelihood there will be of failure in Part III.

There are seldom cases where failure is so marked that the student is unable to perform even the first, elementary exercises, although even these are not easy. Usually, the most difficulties arise with the second and third series. If these are mastered, then the fourth series should be performed without great hardship. In some instances, however, more time is needed for the passage from the elementary to the advanced series than from the fourth to the final group.

The fifth and final series cannot be mastered merely on the ground of satisfactory performance of earlier exercises, or because of carefully conducted advanced ones. At this point, other factors come into play which are hard to foresee in the beginning.

The realm of intuition must be reached before you can be

separated from your mortal shell, while still alive and in full consciousness. Otherwise, exercises Nos. 9 and 9A may remain mere empty symbols. You have to achieve that peace which actually surpasses all mental understanding. Think about it!

It would be advisable to read the initiatory Upanishadic verse, given as the conclusion of this book, and merge into the deep peace streaming from it.

XIV

The Psychology of Success

It is a well-known fact that in spite of the books already existing about meditation and concentration, only an infinitesimal number of readers and students are able to get any real profit from their work.

There are many causes to explain this. Firstly, these books often contain too theoretical an exposition, written more as a kind of compilation from borrowed materials than from personal experience. This deprives them of their living values.

Secondly, overloading of the exercises with unnecessary details only complicates matters and makes the student feel as if he were in a dense forest. The difficulty of ruling our mind comes *just from complicated thinking,* which hinders every attempt at one-pointedness. A mind unacquainted with strong, concentrated thinking about very simple objects needs first to eradicate the old bad habits. If in a manual of concentration the student fails to find the right instructions, where else can he find them?

Thirdly, some books have been conceived and presented in the form of written lectures suited to readers more or less familiar with the subject, *but not designed for practical study,* which alone can bring the desired results. But there is no need for a book about mathematics to be written in verse.

A student cannot derive much profit from a work which, apart from its really necessary exercises and useful instructions, does not form a harmonious whole, controlling his development and leading him from the simple to the advanced exercises, while the mass of theoretical material is spread throughout the rest of the text.

Such an arrangement is even against the very idea of concentrated and directed effort which is expected from the student.

One must know what has to be passed through and what difficulties have to be encountered.

The reader is seldom in the position to separate easily what is essential from what can safely be omitted. He accepts everything as given, and disappointment is the common result.

Another cause of failure is the lack of essential explanatory material, to introduce the reader into another sphere where he can operate under *new conditions* and *new techniques of thinking*. Next, the nature of thought must be briefly explained. The proper attitude permitting success in the study should be adopted, for without it the exercises will remain only lifeless formulas.

It is hoped that the earnest student will get the best that is possible from the present course, which leaves as few questions unanswered as can be foreseen. Hence, in this chapter you will find the preliminaries and explanations, introducing Part III—"The Techniques." This chapter must be well *understood* and *agreed with* before the exercises are started.

1. If you accept and believe that you are able, now or in the future, with the aid of this book to rule your thinking processes in accordance with your will, then two other facts emerge:

a. That you are not your thoughts, which compose the mind. The ruler and the object ruled can never be identical.

Further, the rider and his horse are two, not one. Meditate at length about this until you are utterly convinced of the truth of the statement. Be careful *not to start any exercises* before establishing the certainty of this for yourself, if you want to avoid disappointment when trying to gain practical powers of concentration.

b. Of the two, the rider and his horse—if you like this simile—the *first is essential* and is of foremost importance to you, because *you and he are one.*

We have to be sincere with ourselves. Therefore you have to accept the fact that until you fully dominate your steed, you do not know and cannot clearly define that its rider is you.

This knowledge comes only as the ultimate result of your study, *never before.* But for your success in concentration, there is no necessity or urge to anticipate this solution, which is even impossible for the mind. What is actually needed is the basic fact of the division between you and your mind.

This second statement should also be meditated on after (*a*) has been firmly established in your consciousness beyond any doubt. And no exercise should be attempted before the fulfillment of condition (*b*) above.

As you can see, practical study cannot be commenced without a suitable psychological and rational background. This should be fully realized.

The deliberations should be practiced at least twice daily, the best times being morning and evening—the "two periods of peace." If you like doing them, you may continue for even more than the routine fifteen minutes. An old rule tells us that sunrise and sunset are the best times for all meditations, and these should be used for our preparation. But do not feel concerned if these two periods are inconvenient, as times better suited to your circumstances will do equally well.

The only condition is that these few minutes must be exempt from any outer disturbances which might upset you. For, after all, you are very much dependent upon and affected by your surroundings. A quiet room, a corner of a garden, a church pew, a lonely hillside, seashore or river bank, all of these are suitable.

2. Now you are almost ready for the exercises. But there still remains something which is as indispensable as (*a*) and (*b*) of 1 above. The deadliest enemy of successful concentration which can and does annihilate all the most careful preparations is the *emotional-mental habit of expectation.* It must be pitilessly killed and completely eradicated, for it would destroy all your hopes if you allowed it to grow and thrive.

All the disappointments and lost years spent on unsuccessful efforts come from just that strange and deadly desire, the "vasana of expectation"; of belief *in the necessity of continuous thinking;* of a dull subconscious and false hope *that something useful may come from your feverish thinking.* This enemy is relentless. All your waking hours, during which he usually reigns supreme, *are still not enough for him!* He does not agree to allow you even these paltry fifteen minutes which you try to rescue from his greedy power!

As soon as you commence an exercise, you will notice that after a few seconds spent on thinking about one of the themes given in the following chapters, a *swarm of thoughts start to attack you,* so that you may temporarily forget what you meant to do in this quarter of an hour. All of these thoughts are of no special importance, but the enemy whispers that they are of great interest to you.

If you accept this lie, your efforts will be wasted. The fifteen minutes will pass without any noticeable result, you will only lose time, and the poison of doubt and disappointment will begin to undermine your decision to study the subject. If analyzed properly, *all obstacles* can be ascribed to just this *"spirit of expectation."*

I am leaving this experimental work to the student so that he can test for himself the statements I have made.

Now, how have we to proceed in order to defeat such obstacles? Only by clear thinking and deliberation—which you may also call meditation—*about the falsity* of the attitude in which one feverishly expects and accepts *every thought* that clusters round the mind-brain like bees at their hive.

Try saying to yourself:

"Apart from these fifteen or thirty minutes I wish to devote to concentration, I have *all* the rest of the day left for thinking. There is no reason to obey wandering thoughts, generated and harbored by my rebellious mind. *Nothing of importance can happen if I allow thoughts to occupy this small portion of my time when I want to be myself, independent of all outer things*, instead of being like a rudderless boat tossed about by the waves of the mind.

"*No good will come from thinking during the time dedicated to exercises*. So I firmly resolve here and now that: *I am not interested in any thoughts or emotions during this period when I am trying to concentrate my wayward mind. I am indifferent to whatever may happen. Every intruding thought is an enemy* and I am simply *NOT INTERESTED* in it. I have the inner power to ignore everything that tries to enter or arise in my mind while I am here at this time."

Of course, the words of this meditation—which is meant to precede the exercises proper—may be changed slightly, but the idea should be the same.

"*I am no longer interested in anything*. I am leaving everything outside the door of my mind. I am free from all its usual vibrations." This must conclude the preparation just described. It is possible that you will have to spend weeks on it, in order to create the indicated currents of thought, before it really works. But better to use weeks or even months trying to make the aim (i.e., concentration) attainable, than to spend years on unsuccessful practices, with your only reward bitter disappointment and loss of irretrievable time.

If you persist in 1 and 2 above, you will find that, in time, a wonderful feeling of freedom in your everyday consciousness begins to give you a foretaste of the treasure that is true peace of mind. Then will come some advanced and more difficult exercises, which you will perform in due time with the newly won ability to impose peace on your thoughts.

The key to success in this study is *just the losing of interest in uncontrolled thinking.* With that key you may open the golden gate, from which you expect so much. Without the key, there is no purpose in even beginning the exercises.

Another result of the *domination of one's mind* is the ability to feel and see emotions and thoughts in the surrounding astro-mental worlds, no matter how close or distant they may be. This, of course, is none other than clairvoyance; but not any spontaneous, uncontrolled and vague faculty. If developed as a result of systematic training, it becomes just like the normal physical senses of seeing and hearing, but infinitely more subtle and far-reaching. In the beginning, you will only observe that in some instances you become able *to forecast* words about to be used by the person with whom you are conversing. A strange foretaste of things to come, which in these moments of psychical lucidity you *now see as belonging to the past,* all of which belongs to your automatically developing clairvoyance. Later you will become rather tired of this influx of astro-mental impressions, and will stop them by the well-known means of concentration; for much better things lie ahead of you, which I cannot and should not anticipate on these pages. Any advance explanation of such things may only lead to undesirable mental activity which will take us away from the line we need to adhere to. The understanding of these matters is possible only for those who actually possess the ability and not for those who merely talk about it. It is a curious thing, but years ago when I tried to gain clairvoyance, *it always slipped beyond my reach.* Then later, when the man had become much wiser, the same clairvoyance became a nuisance, was almost never used, and no mention was made of this otherwise coveted ability. It just fades away when a man really starts to go ahead spiritually.

PART III

Techniques

X V

Direct Preparation for Exercises

When you have finally arranged a suitable time and place for your first exercises, making sure no one will disturb you, retire to the chosen spot.

Sit on a chair or stool that is *not upholstered*. Do not lean back against the furniture. This is important for your health, as well as for the proper flow of the subtle currents of the vital energy or "prana" in Indian terminology.

When the time comes for meditation, the body must be comfortably seated in a position which it can endure for hours if necessary. On the other hand, the body should not be allowed to assume a lazy posture, for then it acquires the bad habit of sleeping through exercises, depriving them of all value. *This should be well remembered.*

Do not give much thought to the numerous and cumbersome asanas recommended in the old and new books on Yoga, written by unqualified exponents. They are entirely unnecessary providing you know and practice *a good one,* like that described in the next paragraph. It is largely curiosity and the spirit of expectation which dictate such instructions and attempts to practice them by incompetent followers.

Sit upright on your chair or stool (the latter is better), with the spine, neck and head in a straight line. If you are a Westerner, such furniture is probably more appropriate for you. But for Easterners, the same asana can be performed seated on the floor, with legs crossed, as is still done in the Orient. There is no doubt that the lotus position is an excellent one. But whichever you adopt, remember about the *one direct line* passing through your body.

If you sit on a chair or stool, the legs should be placed perpendicular to the floor with the knees together and the hands palm downward on them. *The whole weight of the body* is suspended from the ribs and every part of it should be completely relaxed. Simple as it sounds, the position must be carefully adopted exactly as given here, and with practice you will soon get the correct feel of it. Whether you are seated on furniture or the floor, the legs should be quite comfortable. When properly assumed, the whole position will allow you to sit for hours without any pain or tenseness, so that you will be unaware of the body. This is all that is required for our practical study, just the natural asana, without any cumbersome and unnatural positions. It is quite useless to expect miracles or special advantages from artificial postures, for such rewards exist only in the imaginations of blind followers. The great Rishi Ramana never recommended things of this nature, and he himself often used chairs in addition to his usual erect way of sitting, which had nothing in common with yogic asanas, and he stood as an uncontested authority for all the best yogis in India.

Another leading philosopher of India, who could perhaps be placed next after the Maharshi, the late great Sri Aurobindo Ghose (who died about six years ago), also never attached any great importance to the ancient "classical" yogic practices with their innumerable difficult postures, retention of breath, concentration on definite nerve centers and organs, etc. In his excellent writings, he tried to raise the inner level of consciousness in his disciples and followers, knowing that this is the only solution to the drama of human existence in matter. His teachings are rather different from those of Sri Maharshi and other saints and sages, but he was a man perfectly capable of clear and independent thinking, and he could not support things which have long since become obsolete and nonsensical in this modern age.

Another spiritual authority of the past—Sri Ramakrishna, a fine example of a great saint, like St. Jean de Vianney of France or St. Seraphim of Sarov, likewise never occupied himself with unwieldy bodily exercises or occult training. He concentrated on love, the highest nonegoistical form, which in its final development makes a man a sage, i.e., a perfect being, like those other great ones who have already trodden the path of wisdom (the Direct Path). All of them were filled with the same sublime love, when they attained the *unique aim* or enlightenment of all human beings.

So it is with the most advanced of men. When you need information about, say, military affairs, you would certainly prefer to discuss it with a general rather than a corporal. I think you must catch my meaning!

It is only sectarian ignorance which prescribes what is nonessential and unnatural, coupled with vanity and curiosity on the part of followers; but never a reasonable and quietly progressive determination to reach a definite, rather than a mirage-like, aim.

It is true that for some purely occult exercises, calculated to yield certain limited phenomenal results, having little connection with an earnest fruitful study, some special positions and breathing may be helpful. If you reach the final target of this course, your newly won powers will raise you much higher than all the occult tricks. And you will be much stronger and wiser than all the superstitious occultists and fakirs.

Breathing should be natural and easy. The best thing *is not to think about it* when beginning your exercises. If you find that your breathing becomes irregular and strained, and that this affects your mental effort, then you may find considerable use for a basic pranayama in its dharanic form. By this exercise you may discover and learn to know your own natural rhythm of breathing, which will then become your faithful servant in many circumstances.

So now sit on your chair (or on the floor if you are accustomed to the lotus position) and rest your hands easily on your knees. The weight of your torso should hang from your ribs. You will discover this is the case after a few exercises. Then hold your left wrist with the fingers of the right hand, so that you can clearly feel your pulse. Now count the beats—one, two, three, four. At the same time slowly inhale air through your nostrils. After reaching four, stop inhaling, the chest being full of air. The inhalation should be performed so that the first *two* counts fill the *lower part* of your lungs with air, sending the diaphragm downward. For the next *two* counts transfer air from the lower chest into the upper *while still inhaling additional air* through the nostrils.

For the next four beats of the pulse neither inhale nor exhale, but only retain the air in the upper part of the lungs. When the next count recurs, for *one* and *two* transfer the air back into the lower part of your lungs, and for *three* and *four* expel it through the nostrils. Now again count one to four with the lungs empty and then begin the next cycle on the inhale.

With a little practice you will appreciate the usefulness and stimulating qualities of this form of breathing, called "pranayama," or if you prefer, rhythmical natural breathing.

This can be simplified if you wish. Inhale for the count of 1–2–3–4, then hold the breath, exhale and finally hold the lungs empty, each operation to be done to the same count.

These cycles should be repeated for as long as you feel the need for them. This habit of breathing should be so developed that it easily catches the rhythm of your pulse, even when you do not touch the arteries of your wrist. The sensation of the pulse beats—which are the same as the heart's—will come much more readily than you might suppose. But do not try to accelerate this feeling. Just *do the exercise* and let your routine do the work for you.

The counting is by no means restricted to the described four-phase cycle. You may even use 3, 5, 6 or even 8 if your breathing responds better to one of these than to the count of four. Instead of 1–2–3–4, etc., our Eastern friends may prefer to use the sacred syllable "Om." You may also do the same if you wish. Then in the place of 1–2–3–4, you mentally pronounce "Om, Om, Om, Om." This easy form of the classic pranayama is also excellent for the purpose of stilling the nerves before exercises.

Nothing more complicated is needed, except for those who do not firmly intend to reap the fruit of a successful study of concentration and who are merely curious about it. They will also reach something, but its name will be very different. We may call it frustration or disappointment.

Pranayama can be strengthened, if the student feels a need for it, by the use of colors. I will not attempt to explain here their significance or theory, limiting myself to their practical application. They are well known and have been thoroughly discussed in many occult books.

Colors, when pictured mentally, have a subtle stimulating influence on our astro-mental perceptions:

1. *Rose-red:* uplifts the energy, stimulates wakefulness, dispels sleepiness and congestions of the subtle bodies. May be used as given below for all *active* parts of exercises from 1 to 7. The dark shade should never be used.

2. *Orange:* stimulates and purifies. Use the same as rose-red.

3. *Green:* helps relaxation, eases tension, creates subtle rhythm in the mind and diminishes feverish curiosity and anxiety in both feelings and thinking. Used in all *passive* parts of exercises, except those of Nos. 8 and 9.

4. *Blue:* similar to green, but less preferable for use with pranayama. Nevertheless if, from experience, you feel it is effective, then use it freely for the same *passive* exercises as you did green, except with Nos. 8 and 9.

5. *Yellow:* more subtle stimulation than with orange. Both colors may be interchanged in *active* exercises.

6. *Violet:* purifying and uplifting, stimulating inner detachment from earthly interests. Recommended for use with exercises 8 and 8A only.

7. *White:* synthesis of all colors; should be used only with the final exercises Nos. 9 and 9A. It is the last step (as you will surely realize in due course) to the abandoning of all physical and mental attributes in your consciousness, immediately before the dawn of Samadhi.

How to use colors with pranayama? Sit in your usual posture and imagine the whole of surrounding space to be filled with a bright (never dark) ocean of the required color. Something like being in an immaterial, crystal-clear colored fluid. Imagine that you are drawing it in through your nostrils when inhaling and allowing it to emerge again when exhaling. That is *all* that is needed for our purpose. Do not think of anything else, but maintain the rhythm of your pranayama as usual. For each of the exercises that follow, I will include the color most suitable for use with the initial pranayama, before performing the exercises proper. There is no danger even in the erroneous use of colors, except that your "tuning" for an exercise preceded by an improperly colored pranayama, may be less harmonious, and therefore more difficult. *If you have trouble* with strong imagination of vivid colors, try placing colored slides of the required shade before a light bulb so that the colors can be clearly memorized.

When at last you are all set with your regular time, position and breathing, place before you on a table, a good watch or clock, preferably a modern one fitted with a sweep second hand. This hand will probably be painted red, gold or black, which does not matter so long as it can easily and clearly be seen.

During the exercises no glaring light should be allowed to strike the eyes, and no attempt should be made *on a full stomach* directly after a large meal; at least one hour should be allowed to elapse. Also, if you feel very sleepy or are physically too tired, it is better to defer your work till a time when you are more fitted for it.

But it is of overwhelming importance, especially for beginners, to *keep* to the appointed time, for the human mind is so constructed that it likes to repeat the same activities at the same time. This means that if today, for example, you do an exercise at 7 A.M. or 7 P.M., the same hour will be the easiest at which to repeat it tomorrow.

If you will work for a week or two always keeping strictly to the same period, the peculiar *"magnetism" of time* will begin to act for you and on each occasion the exercises will become easier and more pleasant. In the beginning when you are still weak at controlling your mind, everything which is helpful is of great value to you. Of course, after a long period of well-performed exercises, the advanced student may feel that he has become truly independent of any particular hour, and that every suitable opportunity brings him the desired concentration. Such a person may work perfectly even away from his own room. And most successful students do avail themselves of every opportunity. While waiting for a bus or train, or when traveling in one, they may continue to exercise their will power. But to try to do so while you yourself were driving a vehicle could well result in the end of this study, compulsorily brought about by the finish of the incarnation!

And now finally, do your obligatory preparation, which should be performed before each exercise, until your mind is sufficiently subdued to prevent its interference with your work through its innate curiosity.

These preliminaries are repeated in another form in Chapter XIV. Experience has shown me that students usually have a lot of questions on the matter of techniques. These may be familiar to advanced people, but for beginners they are very important. Therefore it seems best to give the maximum amount of explanation, and so leave the student with as few doubtful particulars as possible. Some ask if there is any special way of life recommended for an aspirant, but I believe that any sharp change in one's habits is undesirable and unnecessary. The pattern of life should be balanced gradually as far as is possible. Too little or too much sleep is not recommended and the same applies to food.

Alcoholic drinks should definitely be excluded, as exercises on concentration performed when even in a slightly intoxicated state may lead to *serious and permanent* disorder of the brain. *Excessive smoking* may have the same effect. Such habits weaken the will power of the person concerned and discord arises between the desired attitude and that of submission to the habits.

Remember that in all kinds of concentration the most affected and involved part of the body is the brain. Therefore placing that all-important organ into a very disadvantageous position is unreasonable, for the performance and results will be seriously handicapped. Moreover, your health may be endangered or weakened, and if you possess a feeble body study will be much harder.

It is a well-known law that the practical way of exchanging certain undersirable moods with their feelings and thoughts for better ones, is never (for beginners at least) through expulsion of the unwanted occupiers from our consciousness, for this only creates a vacuum. Freedom from thoughts is a *result* and not a *means!* Rather is it an attribute of a very highly developed consciousness born of a long, determined and successful effort. It is closer to the end of the path than to its beginning. So we seek for something more suitable for the first steps. For this purpose I will limit the astral conditioning of our consciousness to one potent factor which acts equally well on both the physical and astral levels. It is—sound.

We know that certain combinations of sounds in the form of melodies, songs, symphonies, etc., have a strong influence on the human psyche. Some melodies are stimulating, some induce soft, meditative moods, some make us melancholy or excited, while others arouse sensual emotions in us. These provide you with an arsenal from which you may choose whatever weapons you actually need.

Everyone has favorite melodies, often connected with his or her earliest years, or bound up with happy or elated experiences and feelings. For this study you need only to select one or two of those which you really like and easily and gladly remember. Learn to reproduce them mentally. Next hum them softly. Then, when you feel some emotional depression, especially before the start of your daily exercises, quickly choose its opposite from your new "astral arsenal," and merge with the melody, while humming it for as long as needed in order to calm and uplift your feelings. With a little practice, you will soon experience the beneficial results derived from such a method. There is one condition: only a few tunes should be used—three, two, or even one song or melody; but not dozens of them.

In time you will come to appreciate fully this simple method of replacing morbid and unwanted astral conditions with more desirable moods. We do not receive any reward when we thoughtlessly harbor rubbish in our astral aura, so why not replace it with something better and less harmful?

We can cleanse our mental state with the same method of substitution; but the weapon is as different as are the levels on which our consciousness operates. Instead of a group of sounds, choose some sentences which inspire you and think about or repeat them softly. They must be ones which you love, admire and fully appreciate. There are inexhaustible treasures from which to choose, such as the Gospels of Christ, the teachings of Buddha, Sankaracharya and Maharshi and so on, which will amply provide inspiring themes. When necessary, recall one from your mental arsenal and use it as recommended for the substitution of feelings. Exchange the mean, useless things for something superior. Instead of senselessly repeating in your mind themes which oppress you, introduce the luminous ray of wisdom. But, I repeat again, it *must be* a sentence or thought which you love and admire, for only then will the method work and bring the richest result. The Appendix of another basic book—*In Days of Great Peace* (2nd ed., 1957, G. Allen & Unwin)—consists of many inspiring axioms by Sankaracharya which can be used very successfully, if you like that kind of transcendental Eastern philosophy.

In spite of some apparent similarity, this method should not be confused with the use of mantras, which operate on quite a different principle.

XVI

First Series (Elementary Exercises)

Once you have arranged everything as recommended in the preceding chapters and have finished the talks with yourself, look at the second hand of your watch or clock, fixing your sight attentively and exclusively on the tip of the colored line moving round the dial.

Do not think of anything else, just dispassionately watch the end of the hand steadily and incessantly revolving. Do not look at, or think about, the watch itself, or about the figures passed over by the hand. At this moment you have no interest in the form, color, make, etc., of the whole watch or its components, only the part you are watching so intently.

Your eyes dare not be distracted by anything, and nothing in the whole world exists for you now, *except that moving colored line*. In particular, verbalization, i.e., mental repeating of words, must cease during the exercise.

First, note exactly, by the same second hand, the time when you began to follow its movements. Then *check the moment* when your still rebellious mind was *first distracted* and forced you to forget to watch, and instead substituted a thought, word or some other kind of mental distraction for the exercise.

EXERCISE NO. 1
Red Pranayama

For the first two or three weeks, multiply the best time achieved in concentrating on your object by the number 3. If, for example, you retained your attention on the second hand for 40 seconds, the result of multiplication would be 120 seconds or two minutes. *And this will be your first target.*

This means that you have to try to reach two minutes of uninterrupted concentration on the second hand. Of course, there will be a fierce fight with the disobedient mind. You may slowly reach 45, 50 seconds, etc., of perfect concentration. As soon as the exercise is spoiled by an encroaching thought, you *must begin again and yet again,* until the period of your exercise expires. This rule is valid for all those that follow.

Anyway, in this first series of your study, repeat the same exercise for ten or fifteen minutes or more as previously decided, trying to reach the two-minute target of uninterrupted contemplation of the second hand's point.

Under no circumstances should another exercise be tried until you have finished with the first one. The only exception to this relates to a parallel exercise, which will now be explained.

As you have probably concluded for yourself, Exercise No. 1 is a kind of attack on your as yet untrained mind by the means of *concentrating your sight.*

EXERCISE NO. 1A
Red Pranayama

This is *concentration on sound.* It must be performed immediately after No. 1, or at your second daily session if you have arranged for two per day. Take a simple, short sound, unconnected with any physical form. The best result is usually obtained with the word "Om" which was mentioned in Chapter XV.

Carefully note the time by your watch and begin to repeat the word "Om" mentally, or even whisper it if you prefer. Your full attention should be exclusively *directed to the sound* inwardly heard. Apart from it, nothing dares to exist for you just now—only "Om, Om, Om," etc.

Once again, by means of the second hand, check your best effort, which is the length of time you can repeat "Om" *before your mind refuses to obey you* and tricks you into another thought. Multiply that time by 3, and this will be your subsequent target, as it was in exercise No. 1.

You may gauge your true development in mental and will power by observing your initial efforts in sight and sound concentration.

If on the first day your best uninterrupted performance is for approximately one minute, you are on very good terms with your mind, and you have the prospect of quite good results from this study. The shorter the times for your first attempts, the weaker is the control you are able to impose on your mind. But even then do not be discouraged. Some students I have known actually began from very insignificant results of only 20 seconds' duration as their best effort for the first day. Then, unexpectedly, they shot ahead, passing others whose first tests had been twice as good. But in the case of these students, they had been told beforehand all that you have read in this chapter.

If it seems to be more comfortable, you may exclude one of the senses in the initial stages, the more easily to overcome possible distractions, which because of your still weak will power, may interfere with your efforts. So, when working with No. 1 you may close your ears with wax, a rubber plug and so on, and with No. 1A you may shut your eyes if preferred, for the first weeks of practice.

There is an important condition to remember when engaged

in this course of concentration and that is to discontinue and forget all your former interest in occultism, if there has been any. Concentration does not permit of indulgence in any duplicity. *One-pointedness* is its paramount rule. Also, as has already been stated, regular times for exercises are most important.

Exercises Nos. 1 and 1A must be continued until you are able to perform them faultlessly for five minutes. Then you may pass on to the next and more advanced ones.

What can be of most help to you at this stage? Everything that strengthens your will. What can delay success? Everything that weakens your will power. Recognizing this fully, try to adapt your life so that you will be in the best possible position while studying this course.

Unnecessary and harmful habits are the factors which interfere with the growth of your will power. So, if a logically thinking and hence reasonable student possesses such things, he will declare war on these enemies and stop succumbing to them.

Do you smoke? Then you have an excellent opportunity to develop your inner strength by asking this injurious habit just *which of you is boss*. If you do not possess this particular habit, find another and dismiss it as ruthlessly as it formerly held sway over you.

I do not wish to imply that without absolute freedom from all undesirable weaknesses, such as smoking, drinking, gambling, moral impurity, etc., there can be no hope of success from your practical study according to this book. On the contrary, you can certainly reach some positive results. But even a champion runner or swimmer can only do his best under favorable conditions, i.e., unburdened by unnecessary heavy garments, and wearing only shorts or swimming trunks. He will never be able to perform so well if attired in full street clothes.

If you do not conquer most of your negative habits, *they will suck your inner strength like leeches.*

Think about this, and make your own decision, for no one else can do it for you.

Now I wish to give you another practical hint.

Since these exercises are not performed on the physical plane, we should strive to become as independent as possible from our physical counterpart. A useful little "trick" follows:

a. When you commence your daily exercises, first assume your normal asanic position described in Chapter XV, i.e., sitting erect on a chair without any tension, neck and spine in one direct line. Also, remember about the use of colors.

b. Take a little extra time and instead of working with your body immobile, try *rhythmically bowing and raising the head,* then bending it to left and to right. Finally, slowly turn it clockwise or as you wish. At the same time, continue with your concentration exercises without any change. or deviation, just as if your body were immobilized.

If your performance of exercises Nos. 1 and 1A has been good, you should feel only a slight difference, and they will continue undisturbed. This proves that the exercises do not belong to the physical plane, but go beyond the brain. If on the other hand you feel some uneasiness during this unaccustomed experience, then attack the obstacle, i.e., perform *all exercises* with the body in movement as described above, for as long as you feel the need for it, so that eventually you will feel no difference whether in movement or otherwise. Therefore, *from now on, every exercise* should be done along the lines of (*a*) and (*b*) above, except Nos. 9 and 9A.

The final aim of the first elementary series of exercises is for *ten minutes of uninterrupted concentration.* When this is attained, only *one* should be done at *any particular session.* So, if you are able to follow the second hand of your watch for *ten minutes,* limit the time of your exercise period to just these ten minutes, and *do nothing more.* The tension may still be too strong and the brain and nerves should be spared and treated reasonably.

Ten minutes of even this elementary concentration is already quite an achievement, and you will notice the difference for yourself.

But . . . it is only a beginning. However, a *good start* is the forecast of a *good finish.* One of the surest signs of satisfactory progress is the fact that one begins *to like* doing the exercises, and does not feel compelled to perform them as an unpleasant duty.

There is practically no limit to the achievement possible with love and good will.

XVII

Second Series

Once the things explained in the two preceding chapters have been fully grasped and practiced as instructed, and the exercises Nos. 1 and 1A can be performed faultlessly, then you may pass on to new ones.

So one day, when you can honestly say that the first series no longer holds any difficulties for you, the next more advanced group of exercises may be tried.

EXERCISE NO. 2
Yellow Pranayama

The accessories such as time, posture, breath, and the talks with yourself, which we call preparation, are standard for every exercise. But now, instead of the watch and its second hand, take a medium-sized steel pin. Study its head from *all* sides with the utmost attention. You may also use a magnifying glass in order to examine the tiny metallic ball in detail, so that you can easily memorize everything about it.

Do this inspection for two minutes, concentrating all your attention and sight and forgetting everything else. Some people adopt a first-class attitude by way of a little self-hypnotic trick, in which they gradually persuade themselves that nothing in the world has any further interest for them. One such person used to say that he was quite indifferent to all outer things, and even if a hydrogen bomb exploded on the tip of his nose, he would still remain silent and composed. We may be amused at this way of expressing things; but it seems to be a very effective one for crushing the age-old habit of being concerned about everything.

After two minutes, stop the inspection of the pinhead and again use exercise No. 1A, also for two minutes. Then return to No. 2. Continue to alternate in this way for ten or fifteen minutes, according to the time you have allotted for the purpose.

Exercise No. 2 should be done until the mental image of the pinhead is firmly established in your mind without any interference from thoughts and other things from outside. This means that you can then see it not only when you are actually looking at it, but *with your eyes closed as well*. Gradually extend the time of observation to the standard ten minutes, and also combine this with the mental visualization of the same object for ten minutes.

However, do not think that as a result of your efforts, you will be able to concentrate on observing and visualizing *only* a simple pinhead! Experience will prove otherwise. *Any object* on which you direct your thus-far trained attention and powers of concentration, will play the role of the pinhead. A match, a coin, even something still more complicated will suffice *when you are ripe enough*.

Again I repeat, the sign of good progress will always be the same: you will *like* the exercises, for they will become something very close to you, like friends, giving you new abilities and fresh points of view.

In the case of mental visualization of the pinhead, it is advisable to create and to use a *black* background with nothing else but the simple object in its midst. If in the beginning, you have difficulty in "creating" a pure black background, then try imagining everything around you being filled with pitch-black ink or paint. Also, there should be no verbalizing, i.e., mental repeating of words connected or unconnected with the target of concentration. It is *not permitted* to pronounce the name mentally or to deliberate about the qualities of the ink instead of visualizing it. If this occurs it is only distorted concentration and you must commence the exercise afresh.

It is quite possible the rebellious mind will try to sabotage your exercise, by forgetting the real form of the object being visualized, in this case the pinhead. Then a temporary obstacle may be created to prevent you clearly seeing the pin. Your best weapon apart from sheer will power will be your constant and inflexible *endurance*. So, if the picture of the pinhead begins to fade from your mind, first try to restore it by an effort of your imagination, remembering how it appeared when you were actually looking at the little metal ball. In most cases this will suffice. If not, then the last resort is to open your eyes and look intently at it for about ten seconds. Then close the eyes again and try to see the pinhead in your mind for as long as you can. The first aim is to contemplate the object's exact image inwardly for two minutes. When this is achieved, extend the time to five minutes and then remain at that for a while.

I am deliberately refraining from giving you any set length of time in weeks or even in months for the performance of exercises. In all the cases I have personally observed, the time taken by different people studying the same object has varied so much that it would constitute a real harm if I were to give a prescribed timetable.

There are a few people who might be able to perform the elementary series according to such a timetable, and who would then become too self-confident and think far too much about their imagined abilities. And when the next, more difficult exercises were reached, they might pass quickly from their former excessive pride to the other extremity of despair and disappointment.

Easy success in the first steps gives no guarantee of subsequent success. Similarly, struggles now do not necessarily give a sure forecast of greater difficulties ahead. So let us be reasonable, mentally cool about it all and strong in our endeavor. Then everything will be all right for you, and you will no doubt recognize the practical value of the method used in this course.

As an example I would like to give one of my own earlier experiences of more than thirty years ago. At the time I was studying an interesting book by the late German occultist, Dr. Brandler-Pracht—now long since and unduly forgotten—from which some valuable exercises have been given in a modified form in this book. Several exact timetables covering the exercises were listed. And accordingly, the whole of the very advanced and hence difficult part of the course had to be finished in only six months, after which the disciple was supposed to have acquired all perfections and to be standing on the threshold of the higher state of consciousness, developed by true meditation and other practices of an exalted kind. But performance alone, corresponding more or less to Chapters XVI and XVII in this volume, took me much longer than the six months. And before I realized that this was a fault of the otherwise distinguished savant, I had to pass through many unnecessary disappointments and grief.

It seems, then, that the only practicable rule is:

Never begin any further exercises until the preceding ones are duly and completely mastered.

The overwhelming majority of cases of *unsuccessful study* come just from the nonsensical habit of *leaping from one unfinished exercise to another.*

EXERCISE NO. 2A
Orange Pranayama

As a parallel to No. 2, this exercise consists, like No. 1A, of the repetition of the syllable "Om," mentally or whispered or even aloud, *providing no one can hear* and so have his curiosity excited by such an activity. But this time, after each separate "Om," you should count its number, for example:

"Om (one), Om (two), Om (three)," and so on.

It would be an especially great advantage for the student if all his time free from professional and other necessary thinking were occupied with the repetition of "Om," otherwise of concentration on "Om." If and when a compulsory interruption occurs, the figure reached can be noted in memory or jotted down on a scrap of paper kept for the purpose.

Then, before retiring, total the number of "Oms" recorded and so get the figure you were able to reach for the day. If well performed, the amount should increase each day, as your ability and will power grow with the exercise. When you note that the figure passes the five-thousand mark per day, you can dispense with No. 2A at your morning and evening sessions, and devote the whole of your time to No. 2 extending it from the five-minute period to the full ten minutes.

The "Om" exercise will now belong exclusively to your *everyday life*. This means that you are free to use it in every moment which you consider appropriate, *apart from your daily exercise periods* in the morning and evening. It will give you much strength and self-confidence, so badly needed in all inner work.

It has already been mentioned that the most suitable time for performing No. 2A is when you have no obligatory thinking, for example, when you are *waiting for something, or going somewhere*. Travel in a public conveyance is perhaps one of the best of times. I myself, along with many other students, have used this method with excellent results.

The next best occasions are pauses in your daily work and these may be filled with the gradually growing No. 2A, so that very harmful and destructive mental laziness or thinking to no purpose may be partially reduced or even completely eradicated. Of course, this latter result applies only to fairly well-advanced people who want to go ahead quickly. But all this has been done by many others, so why not by you?

As a special and timely addition to this chapter, I want to give you an extra group of exercises, which may be performed if you feel the need for them. But there is no direct connection between these and the basic ones numbered 1 to 7.

ADDITION A
Blue Pranayama

If you want to strengthen your physical body and harmonize the astro-mental activities within it, making it more co-operative with your study and less likely to tire from your daily exercises, then the following directions will prove helpful. Any sunny morning, dress very lightly and retire to a secluded place where you can be sure that nobody will be able to observe your activity. Otherwise unwanted currents of thought will attack you and disturb your inner peace. The best time is between 8 and 10 A.M., and the best place a corner of a quiet garden or field, or the flat roof of a house, etc. When you have located a suitable spot, make sure that you will not be disturbed by undue pressure on some part of your body caused by tight clothing.

Stand upright facing the sun so that you are bathed in its rays. Then raise your head as if looking at it, but without doing so directly, so as to avoid being blinded by the strong light.

Stretch wide your arms with the palms at *right angles to the sun's rays* and fingers in line with each palm. When you feel the rays warming the inner side of your hands, try to imagine that the inexhaustible, subtle and life-giving energy of the sun is being collected in them, like a battery being charged. Try to feel that your hands are soaking up the rays and storing them like accumulators. Stay like this for one or two minutes, or longer if you wish. There is no danger of overcharging. Then with fingers close together and turned slightly inward, bring your arms to the front and fairly near one another, slowly drawing them downward till the fingers are at right angles to your forehead, but not touching it. They should remain distant by about one inch.

Now strongly imagine that the accumulated energy in your palms is flowing through the tips of your fingers and into that part of your body directly opposite to them. The luminous current enters, magnetizing your physical, astral and mental vehicles, and as you slowly move your hands downward, it revives everything on its way.

From the forehead pass slowly down until you reach the region of the solar plexus. There is no need to magnetize anything below this important center. The distance from the forehead to the diaphragm area should be covered in about half a minute, although it can be a little longer, but not shorter.

Finally, separate your arms with a broad sweeping movement, stretching them outward once more and bowing as low as you can, before resuming the original position, i.e., with your palms again directed sunward. Repeat this series of movements for seven times at each session.

The process of charging your palms with solar energy may take from one to two minutes.

Throughout the exercise you should think only about what has been prescribed, and not allow thoughts to wander at their own sweet will. We will call this exercise the *"solar accumulator action."* Psychically sensitive persons can *see* the whole process, especially when the collected energy is pouring into their bodies from the fingertips like currents of radiant vibrations of a golden color. The results can be meager or marvelous. Everything depends upon correct performance and concentration while doing it. *Faith* is also a most important factor, and together with concentration, these two powers are the invisible motors which move and direct the subtle currents of energy we so badly need. This should be thoroughly understood.

Concentration, will power and *faith* are but three different aspects of the one mysterious thing, called fulfillment or realization. When this is reached, the *three* coalesce into one and serve us faithfully. But of this crown jewel of spirituality you will hear more in the latter part of the present work, when better equipped by the exercises in concentration, and with developed will power and newly born intuition, you will be in a better position to appreciate what is actually the aim and its attainment.

Anyway, this exercise A has a definite reviving and stimulating influence on your physical body, giving it freshness and vigor; your emotional-astral counterpart will attract positive currents of feeling in place of morbid ones, so that you become fearless and optimistic; and finally, your mind, for a while, quenches your thirst for disorderly thinking and creates more self-confidence, deeper insight and peace.

This exercise, as well as the following one (B), is a visible effort to put the student into contact with a particularly useful form of concentration known as the "I-Current," of which more has been written in the already mentioned *In Days of Great Peace.* Actually, it would be better to study that book before this one, as it would make your work easier, and give you a clearer grasp of things.

ADDITION B
Green Pranayama

Another aspect of inner development parallel to the exercises on concentration and Addition A, is the next one, which I will call B. It helps to revive and develop the higher intuitional part of man's consciousness. From the purely technical point of view this exercise is very similar to A.

But instead of on a sunny day, you perform your activities in a suitable place during the evening between 8 and 10 P.M., when the moon is full or close to full. It can be any phase before the full moon and on the evening of its peak, but *not* when it is on the wane. This should be remembered and the calendar consulted.

Clear nights or ones with very little cloud and no threat of rain are best. Travel to and from the chosen spot should be done in *silence*. You should *not speak* to anyone encountered on the way, and in fact it would be best if you met no one. This can be arranged if you plan carefully enough.

Silence should be yours from the moment of departure to that of return, and afterward when you are retiring, which is recommended immediately after coming back. There should be no talking until next morning. *No food* should be taken immediately before the exercise, or after it. Breakfast next day should be your first meal.

Before starting the actual exercise you are advised to do a short pranayama. When you reach your place, stand upright, as in A, but this time facing the moon, and breathe deeply and slowly. Gaze at the silvery disc for one to two minutes, imagining it as a source of delicate vibrations, gently stretching their rays to your eyes like cool threads.

Then raise and stretch wide your arms, fingers close together so that they and the palm of each hand form one flat surface. Turn the palms to the moon, as you did before to the sun. The arms should form a semicircle with your head in the middle. Now, with an effort of will, imagine your palms are collectors of the moon's subtle vibrations whose silent energy is emanating from that shining disc. The rays will then be concentrated in your palms.

Do not think about anything, but just impregnate the outstretched hands with the moon's rays. Do not mentally pronounce any word. After one or two minutes, turn your palms toward your forehead and let them follow the same path as in Exercise A. But this time imagine that the subtle and still mysterious power of intuition, or "knowledge without thinking," is flowing into you from the fingertips of your charged palms, and enters as the hands move downward from the forehead to the region of the solar plexus.

The process you seek to set in motion by this exercise is just the development of that intuitional power about which little can be said, since it is beyond the mind's activity and hence surpasses the descriptive power of speech. You will come to know what this means as an outcome of your efforts to pursue the methods just described.

This exercise requires, albeit for a short time, freedom from thoughts. But if you really look with full attention at the moon's disc, and strongly imagine the process of transmission of its subtle energy into yourself, then your mind will be unlikely to resist or to interfere with your work.

However, if difficulties appear with which you cannot cope, stop the exercise until—by further training given in the following chapters—you can easily still your mind for the required time.

Exercise B also usually has *seven cycles,* each of about two minutes' duration. Use the first minute for collecting the rays in your hands, and the second one for charging your body, just as you did in A. It is recommended to hold the fingertips for a little longer opposite the following parts of your body:

1. Over and between the eyebrows
2. Heart area
3. Solar plexus (most important)

The areas in between may be passed over more quickly, as the energy collected and distributed is of an entirely different kind, use and value from that of A. During the exercise, in addition to freedom from all thought, it may be useful *to create a strong desire to become more subtle or ethereal,* and so able to fly on the wings of thoughtless intuition. This desire relates to the second part of each cycle, when you are magnetizing your body with charged hands.

If now, in the beginning of your practical efforts to concentrate, you do not feel any special attraction to the additional exercises A and B, then do not perform them at all. *They become obligatory only after Chapter XIX has been successfully studied and its methods thoroughly mastered.* Then there will not be so much difficulty in their performance and you will have a greater appreciation of the value of this chapter in broadening your consciousness.

During your work, which started with Chapter XV, it is advisable to keep a short diary or notes on the time spent on each exercise until it is well performed according to the given instructions. For example: "Exercise No. 1. *Commenced:* May 1, 19———. *Performance:* Half-minute until May 15. From May 16 to June 25, one minute. From August 10 to October 1, two minutes. Since October 1, three minutes." This will give you an exact picture of your progress in the work. Such a diary is very helpful for the orientation of other beginners who come after you.

You yourself must be the judge of the time needed. Suppose that after some time you attain the ability to perform exercises Nos. 1 and 1A for two minutes. Steadily maintain this victory for one week, until you feel that you have actually mastered things, that no special efforts are now necessary, and that no interruptions occur to mar your two minutes of concentration.

After this probationary week, you may attack the two and a half and three minutes' targets until they too are achieved. Then again comes the stabilization of your new power. After this go ahead according to the instructions in this course.

As you can see, the whole thing is simple; but only simplified and therefore effective exercises and their explanations can really be of help and yield the necessary results. The more complicated and numerous they are, the more their authors have written them with their minds and not from their personal experience. Such purely theoretical expositions which have not been experienced down to the smallest detail are without much value for an earnest student.

Instead of the mysterious word "attainment," which should be the epilogue, you will find only the cold and lifeless word "disappointment."

Such is the law of occult training and psychology.

Shortly after my return from India, I was invited to attend a lecture, by a well-known traveler and writer, about a South American state where I had spent some years and with which I was consequently familiar. The talk was quite interesting, being supported by many facts and figures and colorful slides of the country—Brazil. The lecturer spoke at length about two of the modern cities, São Paulo and Curitiba, both of which I personally knew well.

Instead of a vivid description by someone who had seen the flamboyant beauty and charm of that vast tropical land, with its lighthearted, carefree life, I was listening to something like a well-composed excerpt from a schoolbook.

At the end of the talk, I approached the lecturer and asked him when he was last in the country just described. He admitted to me that he had never actually been in Brazil, but had visited the neighboring Latin-American republics and had drawn his material for the present lecture from several authoritative manuals and travel books.

So, where was the truth? The man who had been there could immediately detect something wrong in the description given by one who had never seen that of which he spoke and who was using only secondhand data.

It is similar with all occult training.

If we need a firsthand testimony, we should diligently seek it, since it alone can give us that something which in time will grow into our own experiences, thereby securing our hope of success in the whole enterprise.

XVIII

Third Series (Advanced Exercises)

By now the time limit for exercises Nos. 1, 1A, 2 and 2A will be stabilized at a full ten minutes of trouble-free concentration.

So now, for the next two weeks, you can write in your diary that all former exercises should be repeated morning or evening (or both) for ten minutes each.

If every day for two weeks you consistently reach this stage of training, then you may now read and study the next, more advanced third series.

EXERCISE NO. 3
Yellow Pranayama

After the usual preparation, if still needed because of the continuing restlessness of your mind, sit quietly and do a little pranayama or rhythmical breathing for three or five minutes as shown in Chapter XV. Then again take the now well-known pin and gaze intently at its head for a minute or two, until you are able to picture it clearly in your mind.

Close the eyes (you may also close your ears with a wax ball or rubber plug) and while in complete blackness, created by an effort of will, *see* the pinhead, but *from all sides* simultaneously, as if it were in the midst of an extended field of vision and no longer limited to that of your two eyes. You *envelop the object* with a multisided vision.

This may seem to be a very hard task for some, but actually, it is much easier than you might imagine. The whole thing belongs to the mental plane, purely to the realm of thought, which will be completely and technically dominated when you successfully finish the last exercise of Chapter XX.

Then you will know a lot of things for yourself which I am purposely omitting here because it is *not good to anticipate them.* They must be found by the student himself in due time. Such is our method. But after you have carefully been through all the former exercises, you can create an extended field of inner vision, and in it see the little pinhead from all sides at once. Allegedly, some have made this easier for themselves by placing the imaginary pin in the center of their heads, assuring me that in such a way an "all-sided" vision was much more readily obtained. I do not see anything very stimulating in this kind of approach, as it only testifies to the fact that one has definite difficulties in escaping from the brain. Personally, I prefer to place the pinhead in total blackness as if some one and a half feet before my closed eyes and try the required sort of visual concentration. Likewise, this is my advice to every student of this course. Follow the same method as before, once again checking on your maximum time of concentration or unobstructed seeing of the pinhead, until you catch yourself digressing by thinking or imagining about other things. Multiply the resultant time by three and begin to work toward a clean concentration for this length of time.

The next steps will be extension of this time to the required five, and later ten minutes. The exercise may then be considered as fulfilled and finished. The usual two weeks of maximum concentration of ten minutes follows. In these two final weeks *all use of ear plugs must unconditionally be stopped.*

EXERCISE NO. 3A
Orange Pranayama

Technically, this exercise is similar to No. 3.

Sit quite prepared and imagine the pinhead as usual from all sides, *but with open eyes.* Look before you into space, but without any interest in whatever your eyes may encounter in the visible world. The likely difficulties of this exercise are exaggerated. Everything will be all right if only you are able to rid your mind of all ugly and useless interest in the few objects you may see during No. 3A.

Anyway, it must be performed, for otherwise one cannot advance. As an additional reward for a well-performed exercise, you will make an amazing discovery: when your attention was fully directed to the "mental" pinhead, nonexistent for your physical eyes, they *could not see* anything of the surrounding world even though your eyes remained open and light rays fell as usual on your retina. Only there was *no image in the mind's mirror!* What is the meaning of this fact? It is a very deep, but at the same time a simple one: the world really exists only so far as our senses are turned toward it. Otherwise, the picture of the world has no existence as such.

This is only one of the less known and rarer facts taken from a long series expounded by the leading Indian system of spiritual philosophy called Advaita Vedanta, or nonduality.

However easy or hard to perform, this exercise No. 3A must be mastered, no matter how much time it may take. But do not be too pessimistic: with each mastered exercise, you become a different, stronger and wiser person. I deliberately say "wiser" because the enlarging of one's abilities means perfected ways of cognition.

He who readily *knows what he wants,* and dives into the source of all possible real and imperishable wisdom, can rightly be called a wise man. If you realize that there *exists a source* of all knowledge and wisdom, unattainable by the clumsy, imperfect and uncertain way of mind and its thoughts, but only by a normal and logical process of raising one's awareness to the level of that immortal source, then you must become a sincere follower of that way.

It is now called the Direct Path, far beyond all yogas and religions. The name has been coined by a contemporary sage, Sri Ramana Maharshi (see: *In Days of Great Peace*), who taught this noble path all his life.

The temporary limit for No. 3A is five minutes. Again, as previously, it means five full minutes of "seeing" the little ball from *all sides simultaneously,* without any other thoughts, or turning of the attention to the outer and inner worlds.

There should be no side thoughts, such as those about the material of which the pinhead is made, its color, size and so forth. The only aim is to *see,* to *contemplate,* without any other movements of the mind. The reward for a satisfactorily performed exercise is very great. You will find that it is now easy for you to direct your attention (mind) to anything you wish, embracing it in your visualizing consciousness. Writing these lines, I am also experiencing what I am expounding to you here. I am looking at my wrist watch, wishing to see it from all possible points of view, i.e., from all sides at once. And there is no difficulty at all. But, of course, I cannot write and simultaneously perform this exercise, for the mind must be silenced, and no movement of a writing hand is possible without the participation of some special subdivision of the same mind to direct its activity.

And yet there was a time when the writer was terrified when he tried to imagine such a degree of concentration as described in Nos. 3 and 3A.

So, as the student may see for himself, these things *can be done* by him, because they have been done by others.

In this chapter I want to explain the ways and means of self-defense against persistent and vicious assaults by thoughts of a certain type, which wander through space, or as sometimes happens, are deliberately sent against us by some unfriendly intelligences.

There are both natural and artificial means of defense. First, let me explain the former. An analysis of conditions under which thoughts can enter our minds is necessary for the full understanding of this matter.

It is impossible for any human mind to harbor two or more thoughts at *exactly the same time.* Sometimes less experienced students of concentration mistakenly affirm that they are able to think about two different things at the same moment. The error is that, in reality, such a person allows the arrival and departure of thoughts to occur so quickly, one after another, that he believes he has had two thoughts together. It is like an alternating electric current. The changes of the cycles and direction of the current are so fast that the human eye is normally unable to record them, and sees the light created by such a current as a homogeneous or continuous one. The psychological impression is similar in the case of the two thoughts mentioned above.

From the law of essential and primary one-pointedness of the human mind to the goal of true concentration, i.e., the ability to control the flow of thoughts, there is a great distance. But by now it is well known to you from your former exercises Nos. 1 to 3.

Logically then, the natural means against all intruders would invariably be to select one thought and hold it, and by that fact allow no room in your consciousness for other thoughts, whether wandering aimlessly through mental space, or directed especially against you.

You see, of course, that the method implies that you have already attained quite a considerable degree of ability, and technical knowledge of concentration, which is the object of this study. The method is actually used by men of a well-above-average development.

a. Western saints used, and are still using, short prayers, holy names, and even pious sentences in order to occupy their minds firmly with something which at the same time is uplifting and useful to them.

Then no unwanted thought can enter the well-defended fortress of the saint's awareness. Remember now how you performed your earlier exercises (Nos. 1A and A), and recall how you managed to repel the invaders from both outside and from within your mind.

b. An occultist who is not too religious or a yogi may use a mantra taken from the Western or Eastern books of occult philosophy. There are plenty given by Patanjali, Sankaracharya and also in many of the Gitas of the Indian spiritual tradition. But the essence of both practices, (*a*) and (*b*), is essentially the same. These methods are very effective against all the occasional invaders from the astro-mental planes, which contact your mind only by reason of certain affinities, colorings and by the "odor" of your still not extinct vasanas, i.e., the particular attractions of your emotions and mind along with your unfulfilled desires and passions. But as regards these vasanas, there is a weak point in these ways of defense against assaulting thoughts. It is the exceptional difficulty in repelling, while the vasanic background is still alive; a strong thought directed at you by a powerful mind not always imbued with the best of intentions. If the energy sent is much stronger than your defensive ability, this hostile force will overcome the weak prayer or mantra, and attach itself to the corresponding vasanas in your mind, and so firmly occupy your consciousness to your detriment and loss.

In the first part of this book we spoke about the importance of the suppression of the curiosity of thinking, which we may now baptize with the apt and concise term "vasanas." Now you can see wherein lies the weak side of a man!

In mentioning what may be called "mental missiles," I was speaking about men who are able to project them. Fortunately enough, their numbers are few. All this refers, of course, to those who may misuse the powers they possess. Such people would probably not occupy themselves with average men without a definite reason.

But even against such mentally strong men there are sure and infallible defenses in (*a*) and (*b*), if used with what we call "strong faith." If a religious man uses prayer in the name of God when performing his pious exercises, he adds extra force to his own; although he may not be fully or even partially conscious of the fact.

Anyway, that force is more powerful than all the attacking missiles created by men. In such cases one might say that God Himself came to the help of His devotee, and one might not be far from the truth. Similarly with mantras, if one really believes in their higher origin and infallible effectiveness.

The second natural means of protection is an exceptional one, and by far transcends all the powers of even the most advanced man, unless he is a true spiritual master or guru. For only such a great one can use this incomparably simple and powerful means. In our imperfect language of the mind, I can only call it a complete abandonment of all traces of mental consciousness, and the passing into that mysterious "fourth state" about which the contemporary spiritual teacher—the Maharshi—often spoke.

In our elementary exercises you have already touched on some aspects of the state of being that is without thought. The advanced ones in the next chapters will teach you some more direct ways to the same goal, which is the exclusion of thinking by deliberate and conscious effort. Let us suppose that someone has already reached this apparently distant goal, and is able to live without thoughts and forever remain in the "paradise" of the supermental consciousness.

What meaning would any mental assault or disturbance have for him? No matter how powerful a mental weapon might be, it could not reach the virgin, snowy peaks of the perfect awareness, unstained by any feelings, thoughts or vasanas.

This ability is the privilege of a spiritual giant, and is not at the disposal of anyone less advanced. So we shall not speak much about it, only pointing out the fact of its existence as the perfect means to inner perennial peace, which cannot be troubled by life or death.

The writer has had the inestimable privilege of association with such a spiritual leader, from whom he received almost everything which could later be translated into words and presented in book form.

According to the foregoing, among the natural means of defense against intruding thoughts, only two are available to us, those given as (*a*) and (*b*). In the next chapters they will be enlarged upon and classified into various types, which may seem to you to be more powerful and effective. But there will be no essential difference, except for variation in the form of the exercise.

Now we can pass on to the so-called artificial means against the rebellious mind's activity.

c. It is, in the first place, the so-termed *astral* or odic cloak or armor. Its efficacy is of limited value, although I have heard many enthusiastic comments on this kind of self-protection. I used it myself some thirty years ago in the beginning of my occult training. It was found to work reasonably well against the *lower types of thoughts* based on feelings, or in other words, against mental waves lined with an astral background. The student may note that the Indian classical term, *vasanic influences,* could also be used here.

I have decided to give the earnest student all possible useful explanations and thereby narrow down the gap of uncertainty in his mind, which could lead to disappointment or even to failure. So, before the detailed description of exercise (*c*), we will learn just who is eligible to use it. The *cardinal condition* is that you must have:

Belief, intuitional certainty, or at least the *mental conviction,* that in the subtle superphysical worlds (or planes) of feelings (astral) and thoughts (mental), the only instruments for influencing and changing their currents are your will and visualization powers. In the physical world the *force of pure will,* when directly applied to gross matter, i.e., without any intermediary on the lower plane, is an extremely hard way of reaching any results.

I would like to quote a well-known occultist, C. W. Leadbeater, who rightly said in his *Occult Talks:*

It would be quite possible for one strong enough and sufficiently trained in the occult laws which direct human will-power to transport a glass of water from Sydney, to say, London. But the amount of energy wasted would be so enormous by comparison with, after all, the insignificant results, that no reasonable occultist would ever dream of attempting such an operation.

But in the two subtle worlds mentioned above, will power finds a much more suitable field of action. In fact, it is the *only* instrument which can bring us success. The odic cloak or armor belongs to the astro-mental realm, and even now you can see which instrument will be needed when trying to create this cloak round you.

On the astro-mental plane faith in our inner strength generates will power, which in the invisible worlds is equivalent to the muscular strength inherent in the human body on the physical plane. Nothing recommended in this book can be achieved unless the student tries his best in full belief in his own inner strength. There is no justification for saying: "I am too weak." Read what the Sage Maharshi had to say to his first European disciple:

A man can be weak or evil in his thoughts, feelings and deeds, but never in the man himself, because human nature itself is good and strong.

Those who know their true self do not need such a statement for they have experienced its eternal Truth for themselves.

But beginners do! And this quotation has been given for their benefit. Now we can pass on to the techniques of the exercise of creating the "cloak."

First, adopt your usual position for concentration, and perform a dozen or so pranayamas in order to harmonize and quieten the body and mind-brain. Then intently imagine that you are sitting in the center of a transparent cape like an eggshell, which surrounds your body some three to four feet from it. *Concentrate your attention and will* on the following proceeding, which you have *to feel* is actually coming into being. Here faith in yourself will be necessary. *Breathe rhythmically* and with each exhalation imagine that all the unwanted (if any) astro-mental contents of your newly built shell, i.e., feelings and thoughts, are being *forcibly ejected* into outer space beyond your armor. This will empty your covering of impurities, for no thought or emotion can penetrate through that amber-like transparent shell.

With every exhalation purify the inside of the cell in which you are now enclosed, almost as if you were blowing the dust from the inside of a glass box. This explanation is close enough to the otherwise strange technique of forming an armor from the "od," or kind of prana.

Special attention should be given to the exact process of imagination (which is the constructive power in the astro-mental world) of the transparent and impenetrable, but thin, cellophane-like sheath which forms the skin of the protective shell. The technique is very well known to many occultists and has been described in a few books; but these explanations are not satisfactory, because they omit too many particulars which are not clear enough for beginners.

When you have created your first odic cloak round you, be convinced while visualizing it that nothing can penetrate inside without your permission, and so be quite comfortable and at ease within it.

Then, protected from all outer influences, begin your exercise proper. Some practice is necessary to construct a good shell, but experienced students are able to create such an armor round themselves in a few seconds, or even in a fraction of a second. For our purposes, we do not need to develop our abilities to that extent, as you should never be in a hurry over a study of concentration, for haste is harmful for exercises.

If you feel that the shell has begun to "leak," i.e., that some intruders are managing to enter, then create another, better and more impregnable. But *do not forget to destroy* your odic armor when no longer needed, simply by reversing the process. Instead of expanding it with exhalation, contract it back on the inhale. *Never allow the shell to be dissipated* by itself, as it is not eternal and endures for only a limited time, according to the will power and ability of its creator. Trained occultists are able to make an armor which will last a dozen times longer than one created by less experienced beginners, as the latter may work well for only about half an hour or a little more, instead of for hours.

If you allow the odic cloak to fade of itself, your will power may lose full control of its components, which may develop the tendency to dissolve immediately after you have formed them into a shell. Do not forget this. Also, intruders may learn to pass through the *decaying odic shell,* and so disturb you when you are expecting immunity from them. When you operate with certain occult means such as this protective armor, forces (or beings, if you prefer it) native to the astral plane may focus their attention on your activities in their realm, and they are not always friendly. A weakly constructed shell will convince them that you too are a weakling. This would only be an additional barrier for you to overcome.

Personally, I was never very eager to use this means of protection, and preferred to develop the "lack of interest" in everything apart from my study and practical exercises. I think it is the best method, although others favor the shell.

Everything has its own form of consciousness, although to us it sometimes seems to be nonexistent as such. But you ought to know that nothing in this manifested, although from the absolute point of view illusory, world is without some trace of life. That is why many eminent occultists as well as masters speak about the consciousness of such things as, for example, plants, rocks, earth and so on.

The more evolved the outer form, the brighter the ray of consciousness which is operating through it.

I recall the enigmatic saying of Paul Sédir's master: "Everything in the world has its corresponding counterpart on another plane of existence." And the mysterious Monsieur Andréas went on to say: "A precious emerald here on earth might be an archangel in another kingdom of nature."

All this has been mentioned in order to help you to cultivate a correct and therefore fruitful attitude toward the manifestations of the surrounding worlds, visible as well as still invisible to you.

For example, if you create the odic armor, and after using it allow it to dissolve through your negligence, then as a final result you might well find yourself unable to re-create this protection at all. This is because the components of the astromental shell, guarding your mind against violent invaders, although still charged with your will power, may acquire the bad habit of obeying your will only for as long as you exercise it, thus rendering your effort almost void. In this event, at the moment when you create the shell and its vacuum, and pass on to your actual exercise, the undisciplined elements begin to disintegrate and your protective covering loses its practical value. Then thoughts begin to pass through the chinks in your odic armor, thereby disturbing your concentration. But what is still worse, this occurrence *robs you of your faith* in the effectiveness of these instructions. This in turn diminishes your chance of successful work in the future, and creates a sense of disappointment which pulls you down once again.

So the student must be quite clear in recognizing that every instruction found in this book should be fulfilled exactly as given.

Immediately after your exercise inside the shell is completed —instead of, but on the same principle as that previously described for cleaning the interior—use the short, sharp thought:

"Now I am setting you free, elements of my armor!"

By adopting such a proceeding you expand your power to accumulate fresh particles for the formation of new protective coverings, and the components develop the habit of obeying you and serving under your control.

Other authors attach even more importance and usefulness to the odic armor, claiming it to be a good shield against many physical dangers. But we have no time or reason to occupy ourselves with things which have no direct relation to the present study. The chief rule of always aiming at one-pointedness in every effort should be followed even in the expounding of this subject, as it is the only guarantee of success.

d. The second and last artificial means of astro-mental defense is the *oral one.*

Sometimes this exercise is referred to as the "use of mantras." The theoretical basis of it is:

1. The familiar fact that a man cannot possibly have two or more focal points for his attention.

2. That vibrating energy enclosed in a rhythmical repetition of the same sequence of sounds creates a protective layer round you.

In order to perform this exercise you should begin as before in the formation of the odic covering, i.e., assume the appropriate position and rhythm of breathing. But instead of visualizing the shell and its astro-mental vacuum, slowly pronounce a short sentence which has an elevating significance for you. It can be anything which you consider to be wise and sacred. Perhaps an aphorism from one of the great spiritual masters of humanity, a pious verse, a noble thought, etc. The best results will be obtained with words which find a deep echo in your heart and mind. Apart from the many sayings of Christ and Buddha, the old Hindu Gayatri can also be very helpful.

The student can find a large collection of this kind in the latest edition of *In Days of Great Peace*. You have full liberty in your choice.

Once it has been made, begin to repeat it aloud or to whisper it for some three to five minutes, until you feel yourself well acquainted and at ease with it. But *never* under any circumstances *should you switch from one sentence to another,* as if seeking the most suitable one. If you wish to know the truth, all of them have (for your present purpose) exactly the same value.

And finally here is a recently tested exercise which should prove very effective, especially for students who might not be too interested in concentration as a means for spiritual advancement, but who principally want to achieve control of their minds for utilitarian purposes. The basis guaranteeing success is the same as before: the strong mental conviction that any yielding by us to the onslaught of thoughts which evade control and selection, is purposeless and therefore should not be tolerated. We should simply not have any *interest* in the infinite variety of mental currents which try to affect our consciousness.

As usual before an exercise, sit quietly and try not to allow any thought to enter your mind. Soon you may note that some thoughts, despite your intention to exclude them, still manage to slip through and occupy your mind. Immediately catch the *first intruding thought* and crush it with the firm mental pronunciation of "No!" Put all your awareness behind that one little word, at the same time acknowledging the futility of accepting unwanted thoughts and feeding them with your own energy while harboring them in your mind. Repel them with your strong "No!" just as you might push away a small pebble or other obstacle on your path. The intruding mental or astral "visitors" will be temporarily ejected and you may remain free of them for a little while. But then comes a new one and again your sword "No!" should cut the wings of the invading bird and not permit it to nest in your mind. As the fight continues, you will find that the periods of purity of your awareness between the use of your "No!" weapon gradually become longer. This indicates that your strength is growing and that the intruders are losing their former vigor, continually being repelled from your now well-defended fortress.

Even so, your simple, but so powerful weapon must always remain sharp. This means that by throwing your "No!"—as a boxer does a punch—*no other thought* dares to oppose it. Some students think of this means as being an absolute veto directed against vibrations of mental matter which are capable of being repelled. Anyway, the more you practice your "No!," the more its efficacy and your power of control grow.

It is our troublesome and treacherous mind which tries to dictate something else. When repeating the sentence listen carefully to its sound as well as to the pronunciation of the words, and also to their meaning. For this is the correct way to use this kind of mental defense.

When you are absorbed in it, you cannot think of anything else, and all thoughts simply find your mind firmly closed to their entrance. This is just what we are aiming at. Both these artificial methods are not hard to use, and they do not call for anything above the average intelligence in a student, apart from his determination to pursue the study to a successful conclusion.

If one of them gives you satisfactory results, there is no need to use both of these defenses, i.e., the odic shell and the mantra.

An old rule which can be confirmed over and over is: "Not too many exercises. Just select tested ones that have proved effective."

XIX

Fourth Series

Now that you have mastered Series I, II and III, more advanced ones are awaiting you in this chapter. The aim of the former series was to teach the student the elementary control of his mind with a target of ten minutes of absolutely uninterrupted concentration. But this is still far from being sufficient.

Now we will discriminate between the two main forms of concentration: (*a*) active and (*b*) passive. Both are merely different sides of the same coin, and both are absolutely indispensable. Without an adequate ability for *active* concentration—which is the uninterrupted thinking about a very simple mental image without words and other kinds of verbalization—no one would be able to perform the much more difficult *passive* concentration. And this is the complete cleaning of the mind of all thoughts and emotions.

EXERCISE NO. 4
Red Pranayama

Be seated as usual. Preferably, do not use any of the defenses given in (*a*), (*b*) and (*c*) of the preceding chapter, for this and the following exercises. It is assumed that the first three series—Nos. 1, 1A, 2, 2A, 3, 3A—have already enabled you to pass on to these new ones.

Do a little pranayama if you like it, and feel that it is doing you good. Close your eyes. You may also insert rubber or wax plugs in your ears, if you feel your work is being distorted by the outside world of sounds. This is only a temporary measure, for the full mastery of exercises excludes the necessity for the use of any artificial defensive devices.

Now imagine before your closed eyes a pitch-black curtain, enveloping everything round you. Against this black background, picture a flat white disc like a plate of about ten or twelve inches in diameter and situated about two feet in front of your forehead. This disc should have the appearance of being cut from very thin cardboard and apart from its size have nothing else in common with a plate.

The next step is to imagine that this disc is spinning very rapidly, but not so fast that you cannot follow the revolutions when your full attention is directed on it. It must revolve without any deflections or vibrations, as it is meant to be a perfectly centered disc.

That is all you are allowed to "see," a *flat, snow-white disc* of about ten or twelve inches diameter (whichever is best for you in the beginning), spinning rapidly against a motionless and changeless black backdrop.

Further imagine, and do the same with all the subsequent exercises involving discs and points, that the power which turns the disc has its source in your own eyes. Briefly, the disc revolves and should be clearly seen as separate from its background—which is *the very aim of this exercise*—only for as long as you are looking at it, without any interruptions or forgetfulness. This concept may help you to maintain your full attention on the rotating disc.

Now at this moment there is nothing else in the whole world for you except the white disc, whirling noiselessly at great speed against a black background in front of your *closed* eyes.

For a start, the time taken should be measured according to our former method. First, sit still and try to see the disc, as described above, for as long as you can, until your mind escapes your control and you catch yourself thinking about quite different things, or forgetting to watch the disc. Then look quickly at your watch in order to see how long you retained your attention on the object of concentration.

Multiply this time by three and this will be your daily target. The final aim is for *ten minutes* of uninterrupted practice. This is a *condition,* and there is nothing that can change it. Without it one will never arrive at the final aim and gain the ability which is sought: the full and unconditional ruling of all mental and emotional processes in your consciousness, with a deliberate exclusion of same as a target. It is quite possible, for it has already been done by many others, so why should it be otherwise with you?

EXERCISE NO. 4A
Red Pranayama

When exercise No. 4 is completed—which will probably take you about two weeks—pass on to its further development. At each daily session diminish, by one inch, the size of the rotating disc from its original diameter of about twelve inches. So, on the first day of the modification of No. 4, you will see the disc smaller by one inch; on the second day by two inches, on the third by three, and so on, until you have one of about an inch. Then the next day reduce the size to that of a pea, and later to a white revolving *point* on the same pitch-black background.

It can happen that you may have some difficulties with the mental diminishing of the disc by an inch each day. If so, cut out one of approximately twelve inches from thin white cardboard.

Using a pair of compasses draw another circle inside the first one, with a radius reduced by half an inch to give you a new disc of eleven inches in diameter.

Repeat this operation ten times, until there remains only a one-inch disc. Then you will have eleven concentric circles on your piece of cardboard, each of them with a diameter shorter by an inch.

Now carefully observe the original circle with which you commenced working. Then visualize it with closed eyes, checking the exactness of the mental picture. If it was satisfactory, cut away the first circle so that only an eleven-inch disc remains. Look at it again, then do the same with eyes closed, comparing the results. Sometimes a student cannot reach the desired results in visualization of the daily diminishing disc, and therefore the picture may be confused. If this is the case he should not adhere to the period of only one day for each new size, but must devote as many days as are actually needed for the exact and hence satisfactory performance of the whole exercise.

As always, ten minutes remains as the target for each stage of visualization of the rotating disc. This exercise is perhaps one of the most important in this course, as by its use the student can check his own development and future prospects.

Months may be required to attain a faultless performance of this exercise, but in this case time has only a secondary value: the essential thing is the successful outcome.

EXERCISE NO. 5
Green Pranayama

We have now reached the climax of this series. When you are able to watch, without any thoughts, the rapidly whirling little white point on the vast black backdrop for ten minutes, then you may make the next step. After the usual preparation on a day when you are feeling well composed, imagine *only* the black background, but this time *without a white disc or point* on it. Visualize it in the full silence of your mind, for *ten minutes,* just as you did at the end of No. 4.

If you cannot achieve this time on the first day, repeat as often as needed until you are able to perform it correctly. If you are able to do it, watch the state of your consciousness while merged in this exercise.

Did you still have any idea about, or contact with, the surrounding physical world? If the exercise has been performed as intended you most certainly must have utterly forgotten everything except your object of concentration—the silent, nameless, black screen before your mind's eye. So, although not yet knowing it, you have already made—for a limited time, of course—your consciousness independent of all outer influences. And this is the very aim!

During the experience you were neither asleep nor in a swoon. You were awake, but deliberately and consciously in quite a different way from an average man. A new ability has been born in you, but it is only the dawn of that which should actually be reached. Do not hurry! No one can be better than he is. This is because development is gradual and always needs some definite length of time for its fruition. Inability to perform something at a given time is only proof of this. Have strong faith in yourself, for this is the key which opens every door.

EXERCISE NO. 5A
Green Pranayama

Now repeat No. 5 again, but this time with *open* eyes. First direct your sight straight before you, gazing aimlessly into space, without any interest in the process of seeing. Then again imagine the black background, and on it, some two feet ahead on a level with your eyebrows, a twelve-inch revolving disc, as in the former exercises of a similar kind.

At this moment, there is nothing else in the whole universe, only you, the observer, and the object of your vision, the white spinning disc. As previously, the target time is ten minutes of silent contemplation with open eyes which see *nothing* apart from the white disc and its black background.

When you lose the clear vision of the disc, caused by some interruption or distraction, *you should begin the exercise again and yet again, until an unbroken ten minutes becomes a certainty.*

No matter how long or short the time required for a good performance of the exercise, take as long as is really needed. You cannot pass on to the next degrees until the foregoing have been successfully concluded. The same rule applies to all past and future exercises. The present course is confined to the very essential ones, and no further omissions or reductions are possible.

EXERCISE NO. 6
Green Pranayama

This is a repetition of No. 5A, but with your ears open. And everything referring to it is equally valid for No. 6. You may feel some difficulty in the creation of the different-sized discs without the help of closed eyes. But there is no choice, the thing must be done. I do not say it is easy to separate one's consciousness, even by means of a specially designed exercise, from the *two senses* which play the most important role in one's life, which are *sight* and *hearing.* But when accomplished it is already an achievement of which many yogis would be jealous.

All I can say is that the thing *is possible,* and well within the reach of many of us, if only we have enough endurance and really know for what we are striving.

EXERCISE NO. 6A
Green Pranayama

The basis of this one is the last exercise, No. 6, which taught you to overcome your former dependence on thinking in forms and words. Once again, for some two or three minutes, picture the now well-known little white point whirling on the black field. It should be easy, because the last exercises were much more difficult.

Then gradually, without interrupting the exercise, enlarge the point to a revolving disc of about one inch in diameter. Contemplate it with all the senses "open," for approximately two or three minutes. I say approximately, because by now you know that you should not interrupt an exercise in order merely to look at your watch. But during this course you have surely developed a certain instinctive measurement of time which you can use at this stage. Exactness is now of secondary importance, and if you do this part of the exercise for two and a half or three and a half minutes instead of two or three, there is no cause for concern.

Slowly enlarge the disc again, so that you can watch the process of its size changing from two inches to three after a minute or more, and so on till twelve inches is again reached.

I cannot forecast how many days, weeks, or perhaps months you may need for the completion of this exercise. By now you know best what improvement remains to be done, and what you can consider as a hundred per cent satisfactory performance.

During this period try to test yourself a little: How much remains in you now of that old compulsion and innate desire to think in forms, sounds, words, instinctive reactions, etc? What kind of obstacles still prevent you from immediately doing the whole exercise for ten undisturbed minutes? Are there thoughts about something which may happen to you to-morrow? Do you still expect something from your now ill-timed thinking? Analyze yourself, and find the cause. Again use any of the former exercises which you believe to be most suitable in order to eliminate the inadequacy from your inner development, which may arise from still not wholly extermi-nated weaknesses, or perhaps even from some laziness.

Having successfully mastered the six elementary exercises (Nos. 1, 1A, 2, 2A, 3, 3A) and the six advanced ones (Nos. 4, 4A, 5, 5A, 6, 6A), you can check on your gains in the meantime. You should already have recognized that although your senses of sight and hearing remained open as usual (hence they are separate from the real "you"), certain vibrations in the form of light and sound waves (these terms are used for simplicity and are not meant to convey their exact meanings) were still influencing your brain through the telegraphic sys-tem of your corresponding nerves. But in spite of all this, you did not see or hear anything, being deliberately merged in another form of consciousness, which has the power of elim-inating everything else. Most important conclusions may be drawn from this simple fact:

1. It has been proved that perception through the senses can be controlled by our will if sufficiently trained and strength-ened.

2. The foremost factor of that control is something which we call "attention." Even in normal life, when you are en-grossed in reading a magazine or book, you may not hear music coming from your radio playing only a few feet away.

3. This attention rules over our awareness or nonawareness of our surroundings, taken in all the three planes of existence known to most of us as the physical, astral and mental.

4. This ruling factor, which slowly emerges as a result of

exercises performed as given in this book, is beyond and above the brain's functions. When fully evolved, it takes you beyond sleep and death.

5. If this is so, then the destruction of the brain cannot extinguish the light of awareness in those who have been able to contact this light *now* while *still possessing the brain,* and who have discovered the great secret sought by so many advanced men from the earliest known times. This discovery enables us to switch on or off the physical consciousness centered in the brain, after which the new one dawns in us.

The words of our definitions are simple, but so is the "mystery" itself. Despite its simplicity, its attainment is far from being easy, although in essence it is as simple as the ultimate Truth itself; for the only real and eternally existing "thing" is consciousness in its essence. And there is not and cannot be any other truth.

These few statements are made here, on the threshold of the final exercises which lead us to the natural and unique aim of the present study, in order to show the earnest student which *conclusions and experiences* are possible through endurance in all these exercises, and their final achievement; for such statements have made the experiences possible for his predecessors on the same path.

Otherwise, what ideas and permanent values threw light on their way? And this knowledge is just what permits and helps us to go through all the difficulties and hard work of practical study. We shall hear more of this later when the last exercises are successfully concluded. This of course is the chief condition, just as knowledge of elementary algebraic equations and theory is a condition for any further studies of higher mathematics. Preliminary knowledge is just as necessary in *psychological* or *metaphysical* studies.

In spite of all this, many shortsighted men expect a book about these matters to give them something which will put the necessary knowledge into their heads, without any effort on their part, simply because they have graciously consented to read such a book! Perhaps this is because the use of official knowledge on most subjects is a bread-winning one, and there is plenty of competition for it these days, which is not the case with this particular subject.

XX

Fifth Series (Final Exercises)

EXERCISE NO. 7
Yellow or Light-Green Pranayama

Return for a while to exercise No. 6. Once again imagine the black background before your *closed* eyes. Continue this observation for a minute, remaining thoughtless and feelingless. Then by an effort of will, gradually lighten the color of the deep blackness, so that the whole curtain before your mental sight first becomes dark gray, turning to a medium shade, then to a lighter one and finally becoming as clear as water, and there is no longer a definite color before your eyes.

If it will help you in the first stages of this important experience, you may compare the vision to be created to a wall of perfectly pure and transparent ice.

This aspect of the exercise should be performed for ten-minute sessions for one or two weeks, until the time required for a faultless performance is finally reached. If not, you must work longer to gain the reward.

After that, simplify the proceeding still further. When you close your eyes, try to *see* nothing, absolutely nothing. No more trace of the ice wall or water, only the infinite, bottomless space before and round you. In the beginning, in order to tune your inner consciousness to this aspect of the exercise, you may mentally whisper for a short while:

Infinity before me: infinity *always receding before my sight;* the emptiness, the colorless infinity of space.

I know of people who have been greatly helped by such meditation.

After another week or more, this too must cease, and there will remain only *space* without forms or verbalized thoughts. This exercise has caused difficulties for a number of students of concentration, but in most cases it was mastered in a few weeks, or sometimes months, depending upon the *time devoted* to its practice and the *effort* put into it by the student. These are the two decisive factors for your success.

My advice is: try to perform this high form of concentration not only once or twice daily, but as often as you can manage. For the results will be amazing. Then you will really know and feel that *something* to which a deep study of concentration always leads. And the world of *true meditation* will also open its gates to the persistent aspirant. But there yet remains another still more advanced aspect of No. 7.

EXERCISE NO. 7A
Yellow or Light-Green Pranayama

When you are able to perfect the previous exercise, then the time is appropriate for the next one, which we will call No. 7A. The difference between the two lies only in the fact that now you should train yourself to work with *open eyes,* no matter what your surroundings, and *not just in the quiet seclusion of your room or garden.* At this stage of your study, I can only emphasize the ultimate target of these most important and final exercises.

When mastered they must be done *under all conditions,* and not only as described for the early stages of the majority of them. I am not advising you to indulge in their practice while you are crossing a busy street or driving a car in heavy traffic. That would be dangerous! The time taken for your extra practice as distinct from your regular exercise periods at home, need not necessarily be for the standard ten or even five minutes. We should always be reasonable in our approach to things, and now more so than before. Use every available moment wherever and whenever you can. By now you most certainly must have developed a deep interest in this study and perhaps even a love for it. Anyway, without this attitude to concentration in the various forms now known to you, it would be hard to conceive of any great benefit.

But even now you ought to know that steady practice under all circumstances will undoubtedly create in you another mysterious ability or kind of new "sense," if you prefer this expression.

I am referring to the ability of *perfect control of your outer bodily functions* such as walking, eating, working, transacting business, and even talking with others, while a new unbroken silent consciousness becomes permanently alive in you, *apart from,* and yet somehow a part of, everything.

From its heights you may look dispassionately down on your personality, already knowing from experience, and not from mere empty theories or beliefs, that you and your ego—that little mortal thing limited by time and space—are *not identical.*

All this becomes possible only when you understand your exercises, and do not perform them merely as a heavy duty, a burden, a necessary evil, or the like.

This should be clearly and unmistakably realized. No higher progress is possible from the series beginning with Nos. 4, 5 and 6 up to these final ones, and especially Nos. 7, 7A, 8 and

8A, until you *prefer* them to every other activity. As a master said:

Thou canst not travel on the Path before thou hast become that Path itself.

—*The Voice of the Silence*

While reading this book you can see that the exercises are only a part of the whole. The rest consists of introductory and informative matter which is by no means less important than the practical side of the work, since it is the basis of it. In such a course, we have little to do with the astro-mental variety of matter, which is sensitive to all our emotions and thoughts, and so it is only necessary and natural for us *to harmonize* our own emotional and thinking apparatus with the laws controlling the limitless ocean of such subtle surroundings.

Nothing less will do. And no conscientious author would try to tell you that this study is an easy thing. Quite the contrary! Moreover, for individuals with shallow minds and primitive feelings, the work is simply *premature* and cannot be successful as it is too difficult and demands too much earnestness.

After having duly completed all exercises, you will know many things about yourself which before were not even suspected. And by this knowledge you will also come to a certain cognition of that which men call "the world"; but your newly obtained wisdom will differ from that of those surrounding you. It would be unwise to try to explain here things which cannot be anticipated, and which sooner or later everyone must invariably discover for himself, just as we must eat and digest our own meals ourselves, for no one else can do it for us. Only certain special matters connected with the true and ultimate aim of every earnest search for higher things will be explained in the last chapter.

Another useful practice is offered to you. Being almost at

the end of this course, you should again look, for only a short time, at *all* the previous exercises, from the most elementary up to No. 7A. Recapitulate them and spend a few weeks on the task, which will richly repay your labor.

Take, for example, No. 1 and do it flawlessly for the maximum prescribed time of ten minutes. Observe whether you now have any difficulties with it, which from your present point of view is perhaps considered to be easy. If there are some defects, instantly rectify them. *All* the exercises which you have done were performed not because you needed them as such, but only because their performance was meant to create in you *ability* not previously possessed. Unlike the contents of a book or historical dates, abilities *cannot be forgotten;* but they *can be dimmed* if not properly cared for. Defective or incomplete ability is your responsibility and has nothing to do with the mental storehouse of your brain. So checking is essential.

The next and final control should be achieved away from the conditions which were the most appropriate you could find for all your former work. Now forget about those conditions. Take the "pinhead" with you, in the tram, train or bus, when walking or waiting for transport, in short, everywhere you possibly can. If your traveling time is only for five minutes, you cannot spend more than three minutes of it on your concentration, and so on. Calculate everything in advance.

It is not recommended that when away from the privacy of your own room, you adopt your particular sitting posture and practice breath control. You should never allow people to become curious or puzzled by activities connected with your study, which should always be done in secrecy, for the simple reason that otherwise you will invite plenty of trouble and emotional disturbances. It is always best that no one know about your enterprise. This, of course, does not apply when you are lucky enough to have an initiated friend who knows at least as much as you do, or perhaps more, and who is just as keenly engaged in the same study. Then it is quite in order to consult him insofar as you see that he understands your position and aims.

It is quite possible for a self-disciplined person (which you are surely trying to be) to sit quietly in a train, and while holding up a newspaper, actually be engaged in a suitable exercise.

Advanced students do not even bother to set aside special time for inner work, simply because they try, and succeed, in filling every available moment with that work, without unnecessarily losing time. This does not imply that you must cancel or interfere with your bread-winning activities or other obligations, if you have them. Not at all! Essential and compulsory matters should be attended to conscientiously, since they are part of your fate, your destiny or karma.

It is unreasonable to fight against the things which cannot be changed. The fact that you are in such circumstances rather than others is only proof that you have need of them. Not everyone will be able to accept such a hard philosophy, especially where it touches his own life. Nevertheless, sooner or later one has to arrive at this conviction.

To make some efforts in order better to adapt one's conditions to one's needs is not wrong. But to struggle passionately for something which is inaccessible or nonessential is another matter altogether. The choice will be the test of one's inner development.

By constant and habitual practice, men attain the continuously flowing current on the astro-mental level, and even on the highest plane, which supports them during the unavoidable interruptions which occur in everyday life. There is another exercise which is good for the practical extension of consciousness. Its use is possible for those who have fully mastered Nos. 7 and 7A.

EXERCISE NO. 8
Violet Pranayama

Its basis is the use of something allegedly well known to us, which serves in our transition to the as yet unknown highest experience. In this case, within our field of vision, it is space, which envelops the whole universe, and is composed of innumerable galaxies and solar systems.

But first return to the former exercise No. 7A. Sit with eyes and ears closed, and look dispassionately at the under side of your eyelids, as if trying to see their inner surface. It may be helpful to turn your eyeballs upward as if observing your brows *through closed lids.* Some Eastern yogic authorities claim that this kind of eye position involves more detachment from the outer world and everything else. However, you can accept this as correct only when you are well trained in the exercise. Later it is absolutely of no importance where you direct the eyes, as attention has already been *withdrawn from the act of seeing* and you are beyond its reach.

Aim at remaining in this state for ten minutes. Probably some time will be needed before you are able to perform this exercise in full, as with the next one, which is a variation of No. 8.

EXERCISE NO. 8A
Violet Pranayama

Technically, there is a little difference between this exercise and its predecessor, this one being a repetition of it, but with the eyes and ears open. The time target is the usual ten minutes. There is little more to add; therefore we will pass on to some explanations and warnings. These are necessary because, in withdrawing your senses from their natural field of conscious activity, to a state other than sleep, where you are normally protected by certain natural arrangements, you are retiring from the physical world in full undimmed consciousness, as in the waking state. And this is another matter, having different attendant results and phenomena.

Some people who practice these exercises (Nos. 8 and 8A) describe them as a method of using "inverted sight," directed to the back of the eyes. Experience does not contradict this description, but the most important thing is their successful performance and nothing more.

When concentration is sufficiently strong and deep, you cannot see or hear anything, although the eyes ad ears remain open. At this point I would like to give a warning. You should pay no attention to the possible visual or sound *impressions* which may appear and reach your consciousness despite its being closed to *earthly sights and sounds*.

Whistles, whispers, strange voices, lights and luminous auras may be noticed. *Treat them in the same* way in which you handled intruding thoughts and other obstacles to concentration. Simply ignore them. They are without any significance, and are *not a form of revelation*. They cannot bring you anything apart from disturbance during exercises, thereby slowing down your progress. This is what must be fully understood. Otherwise you may be lost in the treacherous waves of this variation of the old enemy—Maya or illusion, acting through the vasana of curiosity.

These things are unreal and without any meaning. They are a creation of your partially subconscious mind and they are also partly reflections of the astro-mental world, contacting you when your senses are closed. Do not believe in any "supernatural" character of these phenomena, for a clear-thinking man does not recognize such a term. The word itself is not worthy to be used by an intelligent person.

This is the opinion of the best representatives of humanity's most advanced sons. We can easily find the reactions of some of them in the biographies of different Western saints who undoubtedly opened for themselves—although only temporarily—the gates of the other worlds and therefore suffered all the resultant consequences.

St. Anthony the Great, who all his life was a special target for the attacks of inimical forces, invisible to other people, told his disciples that all the apparently "real" phenomena which occurred around and inside his poor hut in the Egyptian desert, although so terrible and aggressive, were as utterly unreal as a mirage. Knowledge of this gave him the necessary power to resist all the horrors and temptations. Another saint of the eighteenth century, Seraphim of Sarov (East Russia) also said:

Know that all these apparitions which sometimes take the form of angel-like visions or vicious devils, are like smoke which cannot do any real good or harm of itself. These demons are truly powerless and cannot take even a hair from your head. These beings can only act through fear, which a man allows to arise in himself. There lies the danger! But a strong prayer dispels all such phantoms. Occasionally praying monks see light surrounding them. *This is also a temptation* of evil which by use of phenomena tries to create pride and a sense of superiority in the careless person. A wise man pays no attention to such things, being securely attached to his spiritual endeavors.

When I was studying my first lesson in Yoga, I came across a statement by Vivekananda to the effect that, after successful pranayamas and meditations, the student may see bright lights around and above him. "Know that it is a sign of your rapid progress," said Vivekananda.

As you can see, there is a sharp divergence of opinion existing between the above-mentioned representatives of Western and certain branches of Eastern mysticism.

There is no doubt for me that St. Seraphim was much wiser in his attitude than his Eastern counterpart.

The Christian saints in general agree with Seraphim in that they warn neophytes against all *photisms,* i.e., unusual lights and visions.

In the past I often encountered these phenomena when working with certain occult groups. The golden halos around certain ardent lecturers or persons deeply immersed in meditation were not infrequently seen; but we always dismissed any suggestion that it was something exceptionally important, showing a high degree of advancement. And time proved this attitude to be right, because the *photisms disappeared when real progress was made.*

It is also of interest that against all visions of doubtful origin there are two infallible weapons—the name of Christ and the sign of the cross. The most simple of people can use them. Of course, high degrees of occult studies may also provide some strong artificial countermeasures against unwanted phenomena. But even such authorities on magic as Eliphas Levy, Dr. Papus and Sédir, together with many others, always recommended the simple Christian prayer and sign of the cross as the ultimate defense against otherwise uncontrollable dangers.

Just how deluding and subjective all these occult apparitions and attacks are, may be judged from a few facts taken from the life of a modern saint, who died about ninety years ago. I am again referring to St. Jean de Vianney, whose parish was in a poor little village in central France.

This ascetic priest of Ars (he is often called St. Curé d'Ars) led an exceptionally simple, pious and strenuous life. For many years his meals consisted of only one or two cold potatoes and a piece of stale black bread. Even then he used to say that was still too good for his miserable body. Although almost an invalid, he made pews and confession boxes for his poor church with his own hands. But inside the weak frame was an iron will, and despite the many terrible visits of the enemy, as he called the evil forces which attacked him for the whole of the second half of his long life, he victoriously resisted to the end.

His thin body lies with uncovered face and hands in a glass coffin before the right-side altar of the church of Ars. Many pilgrimages are made to this last abode of St. Jean de Vianney. When I visited the church I found myself admiring the rock-like features, with the firm chin showing the exceptional power of will and character.

The foremost activity of the saint was the hearing of confessions, during which he was able to reform the most incorrigible of sinners in a few hours. These victories were dearly won, for usually on the night before a visit from one of these erring souls, the modest wooden house was a witness to furious attacks against the saint. On such a night he sent his sacristan away saying that it was dangerous to be too near him that evening, as the apparitions could be unbearable.

From about midnight till the first cock's crow the whole house would tremble as if from an earthquake, and horrifying sounds would be heard from inside. Sometimes fire broke out in the rooms of the lonely old house, which has since become a small shrine to his memory, and even today one can still see the charred curtains on the saint's old-fashioned French bed and the holes in the floor made by the attacking evil forces. Because the neighbors were terrified by the hellish disorders, the mayor suggested placing a protective patrol around and inside the haunted house; but the saint politely refused, pointing out that rifles and sabers would be useless against that kind of disturbance. On one occasion when a patrol was sent into the house during a period of particularly fearsome noises, they found the fearless priest in his bedroom on the first floor, kneeling at his prayer desk while everywhere in the house raged the storm of the invisible, ominous forces.

The contemporary spiritual master—the great Rishi Ramana of India—takes a definite stand against all manifestations of superphysical (not "supernatural") apparitions. He merely states that *all of them have their sources in one's own mind*. Without the participation of one's thoughts no phenomena are possible, although the persons affected usually are utterly unconscious of the very cause of the troubles.

"Concentration on one's spiritual attitude is the best remedy against all such troubles," says the Sage Ramana, adding that: "All these visions are unreal and do not exist any more than do the temporal things of this world."

The well-known "magic circles" which occultists use to defend themselves against the superphysical powers they invoke and unleash during their operations with "spirits," etc., are only the visible points of *protective concentration,* based on certain special symbols and exorcisms known to them. The circles are usually triple and painted on the floor or earth with special materials such as powdered charcoal, and when inside, occultists consider themselves safe. But here the foremost factor is their faith, which insulates them from the deadly shocks of fear.

There are also other aspects to all the ritual and paraphernalia of the old ceremonial magic, which have little to do with the present theme.

These few examples may give the student some hints of what to expect in the course of his final exercises if he is confronted by certain psychical phenomena brought about by the development of new abilities and senses. A reasonable and enlightened attitude, devoid of any fear or superstition, is always the best guarantee against error or misunderstanding, which sometimes lead to deplorable consequences.

Now we may return to the centuries-old exorcism given in Chapter IX. The conception of the "resurrected God" has already been explained, but the term "enemies" or "God's foes" also has a deep meaning. The picture of the manifested universe cannot be painted with only one color, as there would be no picture at all according to our understanding. So the "dark" colors are used to convey the idea of "enemies," being the antithesis of the lighter shades which represent goodness. This exorcism may be useful for students who have difficulty in separating themselves from unwanted astro-mental influences, which sometimes appear during the final exercises. There is absolutely no danger in using it since its nonpersonal character, with its carefully and wisely designed external form, cannot involve the ego.

You have now completed the major part of this course—I hope, successfully; not only reading everything, but also properly carrying out the instructions. If this is so, then you have acquired some abilities which can be applied to your external life, in the so-called battle for existence, for which you will certainly be much better equipped. If you feel this is the case, then it is best to stop at this point, as the remainder of the book will probably hold little interest for you. Further advancement is closely connected with deeply mystical work, for which not everyone is predestined. What follows is meant for those who are. You may recall that in the first chapters of this volume, there were some indications along these lines, although they had no bearing on the early exercises.

The supreme goal of the study of concentration is far beyond its application to everyday life and its mundane events. If you agree, then your questions about *your own true being,* its powers, destiny and aim will be answered by your newly developed faculties. Another exercise leading to the yet higher range of development now follows.

EXERCISE NO. 9
Crystal-White Pranayama

Let us try another experience, which should be accessible to you if the previous exercises have been mastered. This one does not call for the use of pinheads, discs and so on. It is something quite different.

Sri Sankaracharya in his *Viveka-Chudamani* (*The Crest Jewel of Wisdom*), by use of a happy experiment, compares things which actually cannot be expressed exactly in human language, so limited by the mind's faculties of operation. He seems to have come as close as is possible to the ultimate limit of speech, in expressing a very abstruse idea, i.e., the concept of the true Self or Spirit.

He likens the experience of our true Self to that of infinite, all-pervading space, containing all possible universes, which for the wise man are merely a play of the senses. But even the most profound of sayings which may come nearest to the central and ultimate Truth, are void unless we experience them for ourselves, and taste the "water of life," which is simply attainment of the pure, unlimited and hence formless and deathless consciousness.

So here I am offering a final exercise based on the foregoing statement of Sankara, beyond which we know nothing in this particular sphere of study. In it, if we are fortunate enough to be so far advanced, we can find everything.

The commencement of this exercise is the same as for No. 8. With the senses of sight and hearing withdrawn from the outer world, merge into that state where nothing is seen or heard. Many Indian yogis would be happy if they could perform this exercise. Let us be honest with ourselves, for in the beginning, it is presumed that your senses—with sight and hearing foremost—will probably prove to be powerful obstacles. Therefore, we can try to do No. 9 with the help of the physical exclusion of the affected senses.

If you reach the aim even by means of this auxiliary device, there is no doubt that soon you will be able to perform it with all the senses open. The source of power and bliss which invariably comes to the fore after the successful performance of this exercise is too great and luminous for you to forget it or exchange it for something lower.

So while sitting in your simple Westernized asana, exclude all thoughts from your mind for half a minute. Then imagine the infinite, bottomless, colorless, transparent background of exercises Nos. 7 and 7A, but with a difference, for now *it is not only before your mind's eye, but is surrounding you on every side.*

Before and behind, right and left, above and below you, there is only this infinite background, in which there is *nothing to see.* It is not possible to give a more adequate explanation than this.

And now—*expand* yourself, your "I," your consciousness, or, perhaps, that strange "sight" which can see in all directions simultaneously. Call it what you wish, but expand *this* which is just "you" in *all* dimensions and directions, starting from the "center between your eyebrows." This has been found to be a particularly suitable method of beginning the expansion, although some prefer to do it from the center of the skull. You can please yourself. Gradually, like an imaginary luminous blast from the center, *explode* into space. First, grow beyond your body, room, house, city, country and planet. Do not stop even for a moment, otherwise you will drop back into the center, right into your cage of flesh. Then the whole exercise must be started afresh, while your self-confidence, your faith, may be badly shaken by the negative experience. Therefore be careful!

Now, supposing that there was no relapse or that you overcame it. Proceed further and further, beyond galaxies and new universes, always as if from the center of a sphere in *all* directions to the whole of its ever-receding periphery. If your eyes were open—as they will be in the next version of this exercise —you might subsequently remember that you saw nothing around you either from the physical or other worlds. It simply all disappeared, as the Eastern teachers of Advaita tell us, and, as St. John stated in his "Revelations," there are no visions.

Go as far as you can. No one can limit your present or future flights. The experience must be lived. Do not pay any attention to the "surroundings" through which you "pass," if you happen to notice anything—although this should not occur, and no words or thoughts should be allowed to form in the mind. Only the *expansion,* ever faster and faster.

How far will you go? Experience shows that if the expansion, which was undoubtedly initiated under your mind's direction at the beginning, is pushed ahead to a certain point (unfortunately, no better expression exists in human language), the "movement" stops. A man is then bathed in the light of pure, unstained consciousness, and all remembrances of earth and every outside thing are effaced. *Then you know.* For those who like Eastern expressions, I will label this state the Samadhi superconsciousness, independent of all conditions and material sheaths, which still exist somewhere "below," far-off, in a realm of quickly passing dreams.

This is the way to the high aspect of Samadhi, called "temporary formless superconsciousness," or *Kevala Nirvikalpa Samadhi.* You may be puzzled by the word "temporary," but it is correct. No human being who has not attained full perfection, or liberation from all the bonds of matter, is able to live in the "perpetual formless superconsciousness," i.e., *Sahaja Nirvikalpa Samadhi,* as does a master.

When you have duly performed all the technicalities advised in this chapter, you will experience the truth of this statement for yourself, and then you will not require proofs from anyone else. There is no better conviction than one's own experience.

EXERCISE NO. 9A
Crystal-White Pranayama

This exercise is another version of No. 9, differing from the original only as regards its starting point. Instead of having eyes closed and ears sealed with wax or rubber plugs, you begin the expansion with all the senses unobstructed. In this much harder form, some help may be gained if, before your effort to expand, you first imagine your consciousness to be centered somewhere inside the skull, but preferably not in the point between the eyebrows, so beloved by many yogis. In this case it would not be suitable, because such concentration sometimes involves your sense of sight, and this would distract you. It may be of interest here to quote the great Rishi Ramana, who, in dissuading disciples from this sort of localizing of the consciousness, said:

Meditation with the eyes fixed on the space between the eyebrows, may result in fear. The right way is to fix the mind on the Self alone. It is without fear.

When these final exercises become habitual, then practice them everywhere, even for short periods if you cannot manage otherwise. It is not advisable, however, to indulge in them in crowded streets or at busy crossings, etc., until the ability is reached which permits you to control the body's activity and at the same time carry on the inner exercise.

Later, this too will be achieved, and the motionless Self in its bliss of realization will be unaffected by any bodily functions or movement.

The next chapter will be dedicated to the preparation for life in the true spiritual realm, which may also be defined as uninterrupted meditation. Selections given in *In Days of Great Peace* may be helpful for beginners and even advanced disciples of the art of meditation. Through it you will find something which may lift your everyday consciousness beyond its usual level, close to the ecstasy of Samadhi.

Verses of wisdom by Sri Sankaracharya have the power to "rip" a man awake from his slumber in matter, and to magnetize his mind, so that it becomes more susceptible to spiritual flights.

Therefore reading and thinking about those peaks of spiritual conception so close to the ultimate Truth is the best type of preparation for the subject matter of Chapter XXI.

Instead of Sankara's verses, Christ's Sermon on the Mount may be used with equal success by those who prefer it.

XXI

On the Threshold of Meditation

The technical work lies behind you, and after successfully completing the five series of exercises, you should now be in a position to reap the fruits of that hard work.

You already know of many things which before were for you as Himalayan peaks would be for an untrained climber from the plains. You can concentrate your attention on anything, under any conditions, without being disturbed, as formerly, by the onslaught of uncontrolled thoughts and emotions. You are really *not interested* in anything which lies beyond the magic circle of your attention and visualization created by your own will and no longer by something from outside yourself.

It would be a great mistake to imagine that spiritual striving and ultimate attainment indicate mental dullness. Quite the contrary! The wise man possesses intelligence incomparable to that of average people; but he uses it only when needed, and not as an untrained layman does, who thinks ceaselessly all his life and, despite possible fame and fortune, still really amounts to nothing at his death. For a spiritually advanced man, thinking becomes like the trivial functions of the average person, such as eating or walking, etc. No reasonable man would fill his life solely with these functions to the exclusion of everything else.

A trained man can exclude all thoughts, ideas, words and images from the screen of his mind, and can choose or abandon emotions for himself. In spite of all these seeming achievements, they are far from being the end of the true aim of concentration. They are only the perfected instruments, i.e., the abilities.

Now the ultimate question arises in your mind, which has become refined, fortified and your good servant instead of a cruel master.

If this question does not arise, it is only a sign of partial failure, of some unfinished detail, of a remaining imperfection. In which case one has to return and seek afresh for the lost pearl.

But suppose that everything is in order. What then is the question, this last one, beyond which no others are any longer possible? Once answered, it gives us the ultimate, perennial peace, called by Christ the "Kingdom of Heaven," the "water of eternal life"; by Buddha, "Paranirvana"; and by the modern teacher—Ramana Maharshi—"realization of the Self in Man."

To that consciousness now ripened within you is posed the question: *To WHOM has all this work on concentration been happening?* To your mortal personality, your ego, composed of feelings, thoughts and physical attributes? Surely you know that this is not so! For in the advanced fourth and fifth series of exercises you went far beyond these elements, which are so unreal, because temporary. When you were absolutely free in exercises Nos. 9 and 9A, you did not even remember your triple individuality, and this only gave you a foretaste of that bliss which "surpasses all human understanding." So that still mysterious "I," to which all attributes seem to refer, remains to be found. This can be done only by true meditation.

If you read attentively, slowly and with a penetrating desire to understand the logical trend of ideas from the beginning of this chapter up to this point, then you have already engaged in a kind of mental meditation.

The only means of finding the answer to the great inquiry is meditation, which is an *art* requiring much special preparation. The process may be more or less effective and approach the absolute one, which alone gives the ultimate answer to the eternal quest, in proportion to that preparedness.

Therefore, you are expected to abandon—on the ground of your own experiences—the ridiculous and harmful belief that "everyone can meditate." You know just how much toil it takes for the classical domination of one's mind, and how many logical and scientific experiences one has to undergo before the goal is reached. You will no longer believe that someone who has not studied the basic knowledge of concentration, which is the *sine qua non* of true meditation, can reach the peak itself. In just the same way, without studying Arabic, one cannot read Arabian literature.

You are now on the threshold of true meditation, the first condition of which is stillness of the mind. It is a point of departure for greater things.

In many pseudo-occult circles so-called "meditations" on themes which are given in advance, such as a virtue, visualization of holy images, the play of words and thoughts, etc., are only the mediocre activity of an unconquered mind, which usually lead nowhere. Mind cannot be other than it always is. Techniques of writing and speaking which use the mind as a basis—the method commonly used by people untrained in high concentration—are similar to fishing in muddy water where you cannot even guess at the type of fish you will catch. If your hook is big enough and the bait is adequate, you know that you will probably catch a large fish, but if both are small you can hardly expect to land a shark or groper.

When the mind is surpassed, and the radar of your newly

born consciousness allows you to *see* beneath the surface of the water, then everything assumes a different shape.

You are then comparable to the radar-fishermen of the North Sea, who by not casting their nets haphazardly, make large catches of herrings. From the point of view of an untrained layman, true meditation is superconsciousness; but for those who have reached the aim of their study, it is only the *normal* state of consciousness.

"Samadhi alone can reveal the Truth," said the Sage Maharshi. And in true meditation we are indeed in Samadhi. No matter if you are quietly sitting by the fireside of a flat in London or Melbourne, or under the merciless sun of India; no matter if you are attired Western style to suit the European or American climate, or in a modest loincloth or shorts in keeping with tropical heat.

You may not know one word of Sanskrit, but be more advanced than an Eastern brother who has spent a lifetime studying the sacred texts, while forgetting to "render sacred the most important, and unique thing—his own life."

A learned occultist, an admirer of the twenty-two sacred clues to the ancient Tarot (which Hermetists have adapted to fit the key to the lost wisdom of ancient Egypt) cannot be compared with a genuine saint or advanced yogi, who seeks his own inner meaning, without any showmanship and fuss.

The complete course of concentration should give you a broad, independent and free view of everything. Why is this so? Because we then know that there is only *one* wisdom, which reveals itself to the mature and well-directed mind, and therefore we are not afraid that our conclusions might be wrong.

This may be contrary to what others are doing, those who, from the beginning, order you to recognize certain definite dogmas, or to believe in men who founded numerous sects. "If God exists, then we should be able to see Him," said Yogi Vivekananda, although these words cannot possibly be interpreted literally, for the Highest can never be seen apart from yourself. It is not possible for you to become conscious of God other than He *is:* He is the Absolute Consciousness.

Before we proceed to consider the reward for the achievement of concentration, which is true meditation, there is still some further advice which may prove useful for you.

Can you *be still* now? *Yes,* of course, if you successfully worked through Part III of this book. Then, sit restfully and do some pranayamas, first as you used to do them before your former exercises, then using No. 9A, enter into the *stillness.* Perhaps you may be able to do so immediately. Perhaps only after some additional work. No matter! You can only do your best!

Now realize that this stillness, this inner untroubled point of balance, is *all!* It is the source of all true knowledge, if you still need any "knowledge." It is the beginning of Samadhi, which makes you immortal. This has no relationship whatsoever to lower kinds of ecstasies belonging to the astro-mental realm, which rather are confused visions in relativity (as is the outer physical world), only transferred to a slightly higher level. The Samadhi of which I spoke just a moment ago is the spiritual consciousness which is devoid of all visions, and which is ultimate peace and bliss, the legitimate inheritance of all human beings. You may gain it earlier than millions of other less developed men and women; but they too shall eventually reach it.

It is truly a case of "seeing God," because He is just this bliss of the final stillness, that ultimate perfection, independent of anything and beyond time and space: "Perfection which needs no change" (see *In Days of Great Peace,* chapter entitled "On the Ocean").

Think deeply over all of this in order to build a firm foothold from which you can safely step ahead and merge into true meditation. No haste is permissible in this task. Impatience or anxiety is only a proof of the unconquered emotional nature in us, which bars the way to those who are unreasonable enough to believe that they can smuggle themselves through, and who forget that in a spiritual search laws are the conditions of success and the fulfilled conditions are the only laws governing achievement.

You know these laws, because you have presumably experienced their practical application after studying the explanations and performing the exercises as described.

After the final series of exercises, especially Nos. 8, 8A, 9 and 9A, it is highly improbable that the student will care to ask anyone about the cause of difficulties on the "threshold." But, if he does, no one else can help him save one who has successfully traveled the whole long journey through the exercises on concentration. And such men are very rare. All purely theoretical advice is void. Anyhow, there is another way to render the questions unnecessary. Simply—and this is the best means—analyze your achievements: Go through all the exercises again, *seeking for the weak point* or imperfection in their performance. Any advice from an experienced person will necessarily contain this suggestion about "checking."

The second important thing to know is that the *results* of the completed exercises, as well as the *ability* to perform them faultlessly, are by no means perennial. If forgotten, they may *both* begin to vanish, if in the meantime you have not firmly established yourself in the Nirvikalpa Samadhi. If such is the case, then do not forget or neglect to repeat from time to time what in your opinion and experience are the most difficult exercises.

There is an *infallible means* to ensure permanency of your conquests. It is to practice them *in all possible situations*. Having experienced this for himself, the writer believes that such is the last touch, which permits further progress. There is no great difference between the achieved inner strength and that of physical fitness. Both may grow weak if not practiced systematically, *until the ultimate has been reached.* Then no exercises are needed any longer and all concern about them ceases, for in such a person everything has become merged in the perennial state.

As we were told before, artificial "mental" activity, often called "meditation" by the pseudo-initiatory schools and societies, can be of no help to us. In the earlier chapters of this book, we were concerned with the school of controlled thinking; now, when we are on the threshold of true meditation, we have to know something more about it.

I will now give a complete collection of data for meditation, in addition to the already recommended verses from Sankaracharya. This is currently used in certain circles of spiritual seekers, who know what they are searching for and why. It is composed of seventeen short, individual sentences or verses, each of which is independent, although as a harmonious unit they have a definite sequence and meaning.

All these sentences have to be *lived,* not just repeated by the mind, for the latter method will be unproductive. If you are not in agreement with these verses, you cannot hope to use them. But they are so logical and their sense is so clear to anyone who is not completely devoid of the capacity for self-analysis, that it should not be hard to study and understand them.

They are all statements of deeply personal significance, which must be thoroughly absorbed into the mind and thence into the full light of your consciousness.

There are two methods of using this meditation, one of them being intended for more advanced people, who have practiced it for quite a long time. That is to read the first verse very slowly (or listen to it being read, if the meditation is being done by a group), think deeply about its meaning, then accept its truth as valid for yourself. Focus your attention on this verse for one to three minutes, before passing on to the next one, and so on.

Less advanced aspirants should read as above, but meditate on the first verse alone for the whole of the session. It may well prove to be sufficient for the whole day. On the following day, do the same with the second verse. The full cycle would then take seventeen days to complete.

Although many people like this meditation because, as they claim, it greatly uplifts them, I must repeat that the aim of these seventeen verses is very much greater. If rightly understood and performed, i.e., *lived* and not merely *thought about,* it will lead directly to the superconsciousness, yielding the highest experience possible for the man who uses it correctly. The seventeenth verse, if fully realized, launches you into the state of Samadhi. Consider: if you really are that "All-penetrating Infinite Life," at the same time you cannot be in your earthly consciousness. You are beyond it.

The greater your capacity for uninterrupted concentration, the faster the results will come. Of course, this meditation is not for untrained minds, and it *should not be attempted before this course of concentration is completed.*

I. Advanced Meditation

1. I am not what this world calls "me," my name, body, feelings and thoughts, because in a comparatively short time all these will cease to exist.

(Now follows a pause of one to three minutes, during which the meditation should be performed, or the first verse contemplated for the rest of the session, with the second one treated the same way next day. This applies to all the other verses.)

2. But I *am* forever.

3. I am the one who controls all these sheaths. I am above and beyond them.

4. My true *I-self* begins there, where all the activity of my mind-brain ends.

5. *Who am I?*

6. Now I am creating the stillness in my mind. I have no desire to think any more.

7. Now the sky of my consciousness is pure. There are no cloud thoughts in it.

8. Now I am free. I am beyond all.

9. I am beyond my bodies and the whole planet.

10. They do not exist any more, for they were only a dream of my mind.

11. Now I am awakened from that dream.

12. There is nothing around me, only infinite space.

13. I am like this space—having no end.

14. Now there is nothing which can affect me any more.

15. I am free from all names and forms.

16. I have forgotten the dream of earth.

17. I am the *All-penetrating Infinite Life.*

I Am—I Am All.

As you can see, this is not material just to provide food for thought. It implies the introduction of a particular state of consciousness. A person meditating in such a way merges deeper and deeper with every verse, to become more and more ethereal, until there is identification with the Whole.

Some readers acquainted with the conceptions of "super-consciousness" or "cosmic consciousness" so popular these days, may say that such is the visible aim of this meditation.

This idea is not wrong, although we prefer to perform something essential, rather than to speak about and label things which have not yet been experienced. The words dictated by their parent, the mind, are to be rejected when the higher states are reached.

Therefore, would it not be better to do that now, thereby

making the meditation closer to the final goal right from the start?

Success always depends upon the same thing, i.e., the ability to still the mind and through that fact, to be born into the new aspect of life-consciousness. This final process is the concluding part of this book.

Another very elevating cycle of high-grade meditation may be used on the threshold of the silence with great advantage.

For that purpose I selected and adapted twelve consecutive verses from the swan-song of the late Ramacharaka. Spiritually minded and gifted people will find in them a source of unrivaled transcendental beauty.

a. As recommended for all our meditative exercises, just sit at ease in the appropriate place and time. Slowly read one of the verses below, repeating it mentally somewhat like a mantra until its contents become clear to your mind and remain firmly memorized.

b. Then stop reading and repeating the verse, and try to extract its inner contents as a *wordless idea. Know it, understand it,* but no further word should shadow your now purified consciousness: no more verbalizing!

After some practice in this new proceeding you will succeed in distilling the human language of the chosen verse into a formless, spiritual idea. It is hard to add more in words to this important experience of true meditation. Perhaps a simile will explain things better.

Compare the above process to another, more familiar one: Imagine that you are looking at a beautiful flower, memorizing its form, color and perfume. Then close your eyes and without thinking about the form of the flower, just inhale its sweet fragrance. You are then conscious of the flower, but without its visible appearance. Something like this should happen with your meditation on the verses that follow.

Fix the time for the meditation in advance. For example,

set an alarm clock to go off from a quarter to half an hour later. This is advisable because it is not good to allow ourselves to think about time while attempting to meditate. Finally, the last step comes after (*a*) and (*b*) have been duly performed for at least fifteen minutes each.

c. Immediately after finishing (*b*), stop all thought and remain that way for the next five or ten minutes. What may then happen to you? The consciousness, elated and magnetized by the spiritual fragrance of your meditative theme, enters into a higher state, the impulse for which was hidden in the verse. You are no longer thinking about the truth of it, for you are already *living* it.

And this is just what is required. It is not necessary for you to try immediately to meditate upon all twelve verses of this bouquet of spiritual flowers. The purpose does not lie in the number of themes covered, but rather in the perfect use of some of them, as advised in (*a*), (*b*) and (*c*). So do not hurry. If preferred, you may choose the verses which you like best, ignoring their numerical order, although the strict sequence also has its value for the student.

Such a kind of meditation leads a man to the lower or temporary Samadhi, and the enthusiastic pupil, who wholeheartedly fulfills the advice given above, has every chance of achieving the indescribable bliss of that sublime state—Kevala Nirvikalpa Samadhi—which comes when the full silence has been established in you.

May you experience it!

II. Cycle of Meditation—"Nirvana Verses"

1. The Truth is one—men call it by many names.
2. Truth is all there is—all else is untruth.
3. Truth is all-substance; all-power; all-being; and outside of Truth there can be and is no substance; no power; no being.
4. Truth is the all-creative energy; the all-wisdom; the

all-good; and outside of Truth there can be and is no creative energy or intelligence; no good.

5. Truth is all-Love; Truth is all-Life. Outside of Truth there can be no Love; no Life. All-Love and all-Life proceed from Truth, and are aspects and symbols of its allness.

6. Truth is that which *is;* Spirit is that which Truth *is;* Truth is Spirit, Spirit is Truth; Truth-Spirit is all there is—all else is untruth.

7. The Truth is to be sought everywhere, for everywhere abideth it.

8. Truth is ever-abiding within. He who realizes this Truth becomes master of his life.

9. Rejoice and be glad, for within you is the Light of the world.

10. In the perception of the ever-effulgent *one* alone is there freedom, wisdom and bliss.

11. The Wise ever seek that which once known all is known.

12. There is but one Truth—men call it by many names. Above time and beyond space, and free from causation, ever dwelleth the *One* that is *All.*

PART IV

Conclusion

XXII

Resurrection into a New Consciousness

Undoubtedly you feel a considerable difference between that which constituted "you" before you passed through the experiences resulting from this course, and your present state. I remember how, when I began to work seriously toward the aim of gaining full mastery of my mind, there were sometimes moments of despair.

This was because, when I tried to concentrate upon one particular thought or object, others, uninvited, persistently entered my head, as in a home with wide-open doors and windows. The humiliating feeling which followed the seeming impossibility of stopping the invasion was overwhelming. No outer conditions helped, no matter how ideal, *until the inner force had been forged* in the fire of the inward battle. Even going miles deep in a forest, far from all human habitation and its noise, was still not enough to yield me the desired control.

At the time, I was making my first attempt at using the "Vichara" or self-inquiry. Despite the earnest effort of that endeavor, the external impact of the malicious mind, which did not want to surrender, was still too powerful. But gradually the change came about, and later, when the stillness had opened its gates and meaning to me, the difficulty of developing good concentration disappeared forever. In a few years, the obstacles were surmounted; but it was not the same man who sat in asanas for long hours and tried day after day. There are many reasons for supposing that almost every one of the students following the same path must pass through very similar experiences.

We should never accept the notion that "we," i.e., our consciousness, our "I" *as we know it before our inner illumination, is something immovable and unchangeable.* Such a false conviction would annihilate any results and all the efforts of the necessary strenuous work. We are constantly changing our inner world, until the stillness is reached. The lack of perceptible change in an average man, who has not yet aspired to or attained the highest, is nothing more than the morbid sign of stagnation, like the still waters of a pool which lacks any source of fresh supply, and which is filled with decaying matter. Our immediate duty is to change inwardly, and so progress. The meaning of "progress" or, as some like to say, of "evolution" needs some explanation.

From the spiritual point of view, nothing can be added to us by the use of the methods described in this book. If something has a beginning, it will also have an end. So what would be the use of following such an uncertain way? Definitely, no effort producing only temporary achievement would be justified. Moreover, we would naturally never work up enough enthusiasm, endurance and self-sacrifice just to get something which might soon be lost.

This is in accordance with the Law which directs human life. The conception offered by the spiritual master, Sri Maharshi, gives us a different solution. Our core, or conscious self, which is unattached and unaffected by any outer factors, may have veils concealing the fullness of wisdom and bliss inherent in the Spirit-Self. Then the same *Atman* (which is an equivalent

Sanskrit term) becomes apparently limited, like an electric light globe which is covered by different layers of veils, more or less transparent and colored. The globe will be dimmed and not at all luminous as long as the veils hide it.

But the central perfect light is always the same, although in a less manifested state. In the billions of separate bulbs— i.e., individual souls, manifesting their dimmed lights—there are differences in the colors of the veils and in the intensity of current shining through them. This illusion, this mirage of the apparently real world round us, is called "Maya" by the Hindus. From this analogy progress or evolution acquires another, much more reasonable meaning. There is nothing to add, but plenty to reject. From the genuine Indian yogis to the Western saints, they are all doing the same. They reject the mayavic veils, thus allowing the inner primordial light to shine through.

When you come to this point in your study, you will then *know* experimentally where Truth lies. The wiser and better you become, the less attractions, necessities and limitations remain. *"And you shall know the Truth, and the Truth shall make you free,"* said a great teacher in His Gospels. Attachment to visible things, as childish and illogical as they may appear to us now, are the thickest and most light-devouring veils enveloping your Atman-Self. A man who has many attachments has, in proportion, many troubles. If he has one car, his worries are connected with only one machine and its engine, wheels, etc. But if he has more than one, his attachment, and consequently his slavery to dead things, grows according to their number. And this applies to everything in life.

The old tale about the only really happy man being one who was, in spite of his happiness, shirtless, has its own meaning. It is not, of course, the fact of possession itself which is wrong and troublesome, but our attitude toward things.

Sankaracharya says simply: "Attachment to the body and

to all other objects binds the individual as an animal is bound by a rope" (*Viveka-Chudamani* or *The Crest Jewel of Wisdom*).

Resurrection into the new consciousness means primarily liberation from attachments, which is impossible for a man who has had no foretaste of the higher bliss and freedom. In this course you reached the state where you were able to discard temporarily all your feelings and thoughts, dissolving them in exercises Nos. 8 and 8A and actively projecting yourself into the Infinite in Nos. 9 and 9A. So you already know something about what lies beyond your everyday world.

And you know that inevitably this everyday world will also be dissolved. It is possible that in this way you have found your true homeland, in which case there is little left for me to say to you.

The intuitive knowledge reached by the domination of man's lower counterparts (i.e., the triple ego-personality) is very similar to rebirth, or to an awakening from a deathlike sleep. With this knowledge is also closely connected the experience of the *rejection* of some of the veils, which although external in nature are very strong and unpleasant bonds. Just as on a hot day one discards unnecessary heavy clothes in favor of a light sun suit, so does the wise man who has realized the Truth of existence reject the outer world as unreal. True meditation always remains as the means to the above. In it you leave the lower world in order to live in a higher and real one, in which there is nothing but *existence* alone—or *life*. Life in this conception is pure consciousness, the firm wordless assertion, *"I Am."* Only this has eternal existence beyond all time and space.

Questions concerning such things must certainly have occurred to you before you read this chapter. Now you can see everything in a true light. Of course, I have no ambition to try to put on paper something which is beyond all thought and sense perception. So if I say, in the eternal, uninterrupted *"I Am"* lies the whole truth, it cannot be understood literally. Certainly not! This is the way to resurrection.

But the inner process when you merge into the idea, so clumsily expressed by the two little words *"I am,"* leads to the *individual experience of Truth.* It is hard to say much more about it, for details can easily be misunderstood and therefore misleading.

The new consciousness leads to the melting away of ideas of "here and there," and "past and future." All these things existed before you were able to "see," for ten uninterrupted minutes, *the absence* of your former white disc revolving against its black background. When the colors vanished during that exercise and you were staring into nothingness with all your senses apparently unobstructed, then you were no longer "here or there."

So it is possible to do such things, otherwise how could we know about the methods and all the necessary particulars?

The question of real and relative values now arises. After what has been said about the Atman-Self, attachments, and the new consciousness, there is not much left to say, except the bare concluding statement that *relativity* is all that determines the conditions and variety of the outer forms of existence.

The *Real* alone is not bound by them, for it cannot be separated from itself or divided into parts. A deeply rooted conviction about relative and real, temporal and eternal, will be born in us together with the superconsciousness or Samadhi. If a man was a writer, businessman, engineer, etc., before reaching the new state, he will by no means be externally changed afterward, neglecting his duties or committing inconsistencies. If such things happen, then there is something wrong with his "achievement." If a man speaks too much about his "new state," it is possibly only simple mental obsession or imagination. A considerable extension of mental ability, intelligence and what we call "goodness" in a man is always connected with inner enlightenment. But not the desire to discuss one's own ego qualities. It can never be otherwise, for such a desire indicates the falseness of the alleged attainment. Similarly, those who now proclaim themselves as "masters" in the West and "prophets and kings of yogis" in the East are not even worthy of mention. The mere fact of having "disciples" means nothing, because even an average fool is able to find a still greater one than himself.

The old Roman sentence is always valid: *"Mundus vult decipi."* ("The world wants to be deceived").

The fact of achievement of the spiritual status in the experience of the superconsciousness in Samadhi, and the next step, often called "cosmic consciousness" (see exercises 9 and 9A), do not kill the physical man who has attained them. The Master Maharshi tells us, in speaking about the matter, that self-realization, although it does not actually kill the man, annihilates everything relative in him.

The great teacher Christ said the same in other words: *"Be in the world but not of it."*

Such are the conditions for those who come to the end of the long human wandering in the search for the eternal life-consciousness, or spiritual resurrection.

The more true meditation penetrates your life, the more harmonious it becomes. The inner peace and steadiness gradually move outward. "A man is as he thinks" is an old saying. But there is still another, very important meaning. The contents of our inner world or—as occultists like to express their concepts—the vibrations of our consciousness have a powerful influence on our surroundings, proportionally to the force of these spiritual radiations. But if they are only the lower emissions of astro-mental origin, then they can also be morbid if the person is impure.

We know, even without any reference to occultism, that

the mere presence of some persons may create a very unpleasant impression on us, while on the other hand, the nearness of certain other people may be a blessing for us. As Christ said: "A good man out of a good treasure bringeth forth good things: and an evil man out of an evil treasure bringeth forth evil things."

Therefore, to the measure that peace and bliss permeate your life, so you become a center of peaceful and blissful radiations for your surroundings. No one can ever know about it, often not even the man himself who is actually producing good from his own radiant aura.

No matter! The fact itself is the thing which counts. The spiritual influence of a master, i.e., a perfect man, is without any comparison and beyond all admiration.

The writer experienced this for himself, although he first contacted his master with a somewhat skeptical attitude because of certain descriptions which he had encountered long ago in books as well as from certain personal accounts.

The reality rendered all of them superfluous. And now I know why! Spiritual truth cannot be presented adequately in words. The presence of a great being immediately establishes the subtle atmosphere of the silence, that so eagerly and sometimes desperately sought silence of the full and perennial inner peace.

In the rays of a spiritual sun, which have their source in a true master, all the good seeds in a man begin to germinate and rapidly grow into mature plants.

For many years the writer worked at the practical study of concentration and meditation, as given in this volume. The exercises were strictly performed and repeated as necessary. The moments of full peace came in due time. Further steps ahead were quite clear; but *the effort,* as always in such cases, *was still needed* for the perfecting of the most advanced exercises. So at last the writer came to his master, recognizing that without the master there cannot be any Direct Path to the ultimate aim.

The first day at the feet of the guru was the *last for all exercises;* but not because they were or had become unnecessary. I believe it to have been just the opposite. The ability to restrain the mind in the presence of the guru may be one of the deciding factors for receiving from the master initiation in silence, which is the highest one.

Study of this kind will never be frustrated, but will be only a welcome help in all the opportunities for inner progress. It is a well-known fact that undeveloped people cannot even recognize the presence of a true master, but remain blind to his spiritual beauty, or are even hostile (as witness the story of Christ).

The master can so strongly influence the still latent abilities in his true devotees, that what before seemed to be very hard becomes child's play.

So we may see the position of Truth. But *to encounter a true spiritual master* in his earthly life is a chance, speaking practically, on which no reasonable person *can ever count.* Simply because the great sages come on earth so very seldom, and then only after long periods of time. But the spiritual inheritance of each true teacher is never lost, and even the passage of thousands of years cannot diminish the power and beauty of the Truth as taught by the Christ and Buddha. Here again, *the better we are prepared,* the more profit and realization we can take from the teachings of the masters. Therefore, again the preparation is of the utmost importance. That is why this book has been written. For, "when the disciple is ripe, the master appears," although not always in physical form.

In addition to the technical studies, the moral side (heart) cannot be underestimated. We cannot hope to get any profit from all these exercises if we are still torn by envy, anger, greed, jealousy, the desire for lower pleasures, pride, etc. Why?

Many good reasons exist for such a statement, but we will mention only the most important ones.

Firstly: If we have evil intentions and desires, we are simply weaklings from the spiritual point of view. We then lack the inner force which pushes a man through the most difficult exercises and study. Consequently, how can you expect a weak person—who, because he cannot dominate his most primitive passions, is an emotional slave of the physical and astral senses—to *endure* throughout the whole of this course?

Secondly: There are forces which resist human efforts to grow stronger and thereby become rulers of certain entities of the lower sort, not necessarily visible to the normal human physical eye. If there is not enough firm, moral strength in a man, these forces will bar his way, sending him *one temptation after another,* thus delaying his exercises and reducing the time spent on them. The results will be nil. (Read the famous *Thaïs* by Anatole France.)

Thirdly: Everyone who begins such inner effort can do little without aid from both inside and out. Here I cannot enter into more detail, because it would be unnecessary and premature for unsuccessful students, and superfluous for those who are ripe enough to get that help and with it happily conclude the whole task of resurrection. This help is *not given* to those who seem to possess little or no guarantee of pure aims and proper use of the power when obtained.

Some might say: "Well, but the so-called black magicians, i.e., men using certain occult powers for their egoistic (which means evil) aims, must also possess a considerable ability of concentration." Yes! But they too have been aided, although *not by the powers of light.* Every picture is composed of light and dark colors, as already mentioned in Chapter IX. We cannot paint a picture with only one color. This is to say that there are forces which oppose human progress, leading men on wide sidepaths. We call them evil. Evil is not real, as it is not permanent, being only the negation, the absence, of good, of Truth. But look attentively at the present world and you can see for yourself whether or not it is living strictly in accordance with good reason. (Or perhaps there is something different?) The illusion can be mistaken for reality. Therefore the evil exists and acts. It is our own duty to decide on which side we are and want to be. Light or shadow!

One thing is certain: there is the hope of progress, spiritualization and attainment of the final peace and bliss; but only on the *right* side of things. I do not even wish to guess at the kind of hope and "reward" which might exist on the left, or black side.

The very process of spiritual resurrection of man is as real as every other happening in the surrounding outer world, which is something no average man would contest. In fact, for the person affected, that process is much more real than anything else, for it and its effects are *truly permanent,* and not relative and temporary as is all the rest of the world around us.

Often the spiritualization of man is called a "mysterious process." Nothing is further from the truth. Observed by a layman—which very seldom happens—the outward manifestations of these changes can really appear to such an untrained observer as something inexplicable and unusual and hence "mysterious." But in truth, and for the person concerned, there is nothing mysterious or inexplicable. For him, on the contrary, there is an immensely intensified clarity of consciousness, based on his full inner freedom, won through domination of the mind's processes.

I will make another attempt to convey in words what so easily eludes all such attempts.

To what can spiritualization be likened? It seems that if we accept the so-called "normal" consciousness of the average man as a basis, the process of inner resurrection into spirituality might be likened to that of *distillation,* by which the awareness becomes more and more ethereal, and less and less attached to the former gross vasanas.

Interest in these vasanas, desires, material pleasures and other egoistic qualities in man, gradually vanishes. This point is most important, as it is not beyond mental understanding, which is the only tool of cognition for so many of us. It may be interesting to mention the chief *inner obstacle* which usually bars the way to the highest peaks in us. It is that strange fear of the "insufficient manifestation of life," allegedly accompanying the process of "distillation." Man is then simply afraid that he might "lose himself" in the rarefied atmosphere of spirit, and that there will be little or nothing left of him from his self-awareness and self-assertion.

This obstacle has barred and even closed the path to many otherwise able aspirants, who were not lucky enough to get authoritative advice at the right time, to show that these fears are futile, unreal and hence groundless. It is similar to the situation of an inexperienced diver, who instinctively feels a fear of crushing his body by the impact of the water after a leap from a high springboard. But after a few dives, the fear disappears.

And this is what our diver-student must know well if he wants to make any real progress, now that he has been advised about inner difficulties and the methods of overcoming them. It is recommended that he again read some of the chapters of Parts II and III of this work.

The process of "resurrection" to the new life, i.e., realization or spiritualization of man, bring *no danger* to his earthly life, as can easily happen from unreasonable and unnecessary occult practices based on the human vices of curiosity, thirst for power over others, pride, greed and other lower desires.

It is as if, after leaping into the air from ground level for as high as you could, you always landed upright on your legs without harm.

When using gymnastic equipment, such as vaulting poles, parallel bars, high ladders, heavy weights, springboards, etc., you never have any guarantee that a leap or lifting of weights will not break the natural resistance of your organs, muscles or bones. But no one has ever harmed himself while performing the simple and safe, but power-giving and reasonable exercises of concentration.

On the other hand, many have perished, first morally and mentally, and later physically, or done irreparable harm to themselves by certain artificial methods of breathing, cumbersome and unnatural postures and unnecessary attempts to interfere with the spinal nerve centers and certain glands and organs in their bodies.

May the student always be fully aware of all that has just been said.

There is another possibility for men who strive high. The student possibly sees that this course has the characteristic of logical gradation in exposition and attainment. From the easiest and elementary efforts a man is led to more and more difficult exercises. Accordingly, his powers may grow, and at the end of his study he will probably be much stronger and wiser than he was before.

Some will ask: "Is it the *only* way?" The honest answer will be: "No, not the only one." *What then?* I would like to mention here only two of the principal paths, as they are of great importance and usefulness. All others have a minor meaning or are seldom used; but at their end, all of them must come, although, of course, very much later, to the same ultimate point—Wisdom.

The *first* is the path of true religious devotion. On it man also uses his powers of concentration. For without them, *no path* can be followed. In this case, concentration is rather one-sided, as it only works in one direction, that of religious denominations. We spoke about this in Chapter IX. The aim of such an aspirant is God Himself, no matter what his concept of the Supreme Being is. This path was clearly indicated by the great Rishi Ramana as suitable for those who are unable to follow the Direct Path.

"They dedicate every feeling, thought and deed to God, and at the end they become united with the object of their adoration. Surrendering everything to Him, they receive everything from Him."

This path has many subdivisions, and some Indian Yogas also belong to it, such as Bhakti Yoga (devotion), Mantra Yoga (repetition of God's names) and, in part, Laya Yoga (ritual). Progress depends upon the degree of the man's surrender and the purity of his intentions.

The *second,* properly speaking, is not a Yoga at all, but it is sometimes called Maha Yoga or Great Yoga. Its beginning has much in common with the Jnani Yoga (that of Wisdom), which is therefore often confused with the true Maha Yoga. But the former is only a part of the latter.

This Direct Path has only one aim—self-knowledge, or as its contemporary master—the Maharshi—used to say: the *realization of the self in man.* This means the experiential wisdom of one's own true being and meaning, not any theoretical exposition or belief.

Actually, no true achievement is possible without this condition, i.e., self-realization. In this course of concentration we saw that at the end the same eternal inquiry appears and has to be solved with the new powers gained through the study and conquest of the ego in man. This means a much greater chance of success.

The Direct Path uses nothing more than the basic self-inquiry or "Vichara" (*"Who am I?"*). No special breathing, postures or mental exercises are indicated, although the inquiry itself demands great powers of concentration. The character of the Vichara deprives the Direct Path of any yogic aspects. Here there are no gradual steps forward with different methods and means for each degree or series of exercises.

One thing is valid from beginning to end: the self-inquiry matures the man's consciousness, cleanses it of sin, raises and —in the final stage—merges it into the ocean of the unique, great Self, which people call variously God, Nirvana, Heaven, Salvation, Paradise and so on.

The most useful knowledge for a human being is, as the famous and wise ascetic Thomas à Kempis used to say, self-knowledge and the suppression of the lower ego-self in man, which is now frequently termed the "personality" of "individuality."

A man can be virtuous—which is not so uncommon—but if he does not know his own origin, nature and aim of existence, are his virtues then so firm and durable? It is recognized that men instinctively seek their supreme good, which at times they perceive. In man, the highest good is that which is most lasting and represents his true nature and not merely the outer perishable sheaths.

This can be—and *is*—only his real "I," not a combination of physical, astral and mental counterparts, of name, nationality and race, but *something* which survives all of these.

For a beginning, if you pronounce, with closed eyes, *"I," "I am,"* without thinking, but rather forgetting your outer form, sex, position and so on *then you may get some idea* of what is sought in self-inquiry. This *deep insight* is impossible without certain powers of concentration and cleansing the mind of all its "compulsory" activities. So once again, we come to the *inevitable art of concentration.* One simply cannot do anything without it!

Comparatively few men follow this path, so difficult despite its simplicity. It lacks all the paraphernalia connected with the lower degrees of attainment, as in Yoga and ordinary saintship. *All* effort is directed straight ahead and above; as a result, all the intermediary means, neglected in the beginning, become easy and can be conquered without any battle.

The difference is that on all other paths you try to reach the goal from below, being compelled to climb all the steps to the summit. On the Direct Path, you approach from above, from high spiritual flight, and what lies below the target holds very little interest for you. This is only an attempt to present the invisible and intangible in graphic form, which we cannot expect to be exact, since we are trying to describe the indescribable.

Indeed, when deep meditation on the Vichara theme takes place, a man's breath stops for the period of deepest immersion in the Self-Spirit. This happens only so far as these experiences are *spontaneous and rare,* instead of controllable and *permanent.* In the latter instance, these symptoms disappear, and man can enjoy full spiritual consciousness or the high form of Samadhi, with no visible changes in his bodily processes. This is a very important fact. As you can see, the yogic practices are inverted here. I do not believe too much in the Hindu fakirs and yogis who pretend to stop their breath deliberately in order to enter Samadhi, although I have practical knowledge of the methods of controlling the pulse to stop, slow or accelerate it. According to medical science, breath is considered to be so intimately connected with the body's life that the two are inseparable.

But experience proves differently. By "deep diving" into meditation, the inner stillness seems to overflow everything and take care of the body's new state of existence, and no movement can disturb that peace of the silence. It is resurrection again!

Self-inquiry finds no answer in any kind of speech or thought. Therefore, while he is experiencing it no one can ever reply and explain exactly who he is, although after his experience of the superconsciousness, which is self-realization, such a man *really knows*.

The only answer which can be obtained is that it is a state of spiritual freedom from all limitations of the ego-personality, i.e., the so-called "egoless state." You may compare this with exercise No. 9A from Chapter XX, the "expansion" of the mind's consciousness into a supermental experience.

If *every spiritual path needs a master* or an ideal which can lead the aspirant through the darkness and uncertainty of the first steps, then for the Direct Path this necessity for a master is an absolute condition. At the present time, since the passing away of the actual master of the Direct Path—Sri Maharshi—any physical encounter is of course out of the question. No matter, for the spiritual one remains as intact as it was before.

Since the whole search on this path belongs to the inner, spiritual (but not astro-mental) world, so the encountering of the master in this way is *a reality and a certainty*, providing the search is a genuine one. According to the Maharshi's words, the chief obstacle is "your wandering mind and per-verted ways of life," which means only the lack of concentra-tion in the wider sense of the word.

Many thousands of men have spent some time in the pres-ence of the Direct Path's master; but how many of them actu-ally benefited from the contact? How many became "that seed fallen on the good soil"?

The majority soon forgot the bliss and happiness they spon-taneously experienced on seeing the master. Then, later they continued their former materialistic and egoistic ways of a life full of attachments. The seed had fallen on stony ground!

There is another use for the power of concentration. It is quite possible that if you do pursue the exercises of Part III right to the end, and if you learn the practical secret of excluding the senses from your consciousness (I cannot speak more of the details, which should be discovered for yourself), then you may be able to hear and to see things usually closed to the average man.

For when one's attention is closed to the outer world, a kind of subtle silence arises within. It may then happen that influence from the planes neighboring the physical, that is, those of the astro-mental worlds, can contact the subtle and usually dormant senses in man.

In such a case one may become conscious of certain kinds of visions and unearthly sounds and odors, etc. In our study, these phenomena should be avoided as carefully as were all the other intruders with which the student fought in the first series of exercises (Chapters XV–XXI). These are the things which are so eagerly sought after by many occultists of the lower kind, who are devoured by the dangerous vice of curiosity, as well as by the lack of any firm inner strength of character.

Sometimes these people try to find justication for their activities by claiming that their search for unknown powers is based on the noble desire "to help suffering humanity." I presume that most of my readers will be astute enough to detect the old sin of hypocrisy in such a claim.

The thing being sought by these prospective benefactors of humanity is first and foremost the satisfaction of their own curiosity and the opportunity of using the new "knowledge" for their own private ends. Whoever is unable to help his surroundings *within the compass of his present means and abilities* will be still less likely to achieve anything if he ever obtains some psychical powers and apparently gains control over some astral monsters. This is the plain truth.

There are organizations whose members spend their free evenings on "meditations" in order to cure or help other people. It costs them nothing, and they like to be praised for their wonderful (though imaginary) activities in behalf of human welfare.

By now you must certainly have a clear idea what meditation *is,* and by whom and at what cost it may be made. You know how much effort is needed in order even to approach the spiritual realm, after rejection of the astro-mental chains. And you certainly know just *who* is entitled to speak about spirituality. Certainly not those who sleep or knit at "spiritual" meetings of all kinds because they have too much spare time on their hands.

If some types of clairvoyance or clairaudience occur to an earnest disciple of the Direct Path, he will pass over them just as he passed by the nuisances of the outer world, which try to prevent him merging into the Real in himself, and thereby become aware of the whole Reality—the *One Self.*

For everything which distracts him on the path is his enemy. And for an advanced student, the best weapon against the enemy's obstacles is to *forget* all about them, and not feed them with his own energy, which in this case takes the form of attention.

In order to be able to do this, the very *interest* in outer things must disappear. Then you will always be in the victor's camp.

The Direct Path has foremost need of the master, whose example and grace alone can help us to overcome the difficulties of its unique way. The master does not need to appear to his disciple in physical form. His words and the descriptions of those who knew such a guru, and perhaps even his pictures, serve just as well for a ripe soul ready to accept the toil and strain ahead.

Usually the process occurs differently. Often a man does not know much about the doctrine, when something *inside him* exerts an irresistible attraction. This something is beyond all mental affinities and smooth expositions. One simply *knows,* and that is all. "And you shall know the Truth and the Truth shall make you free." Under the tuition of a genuine master, all the dangers of this strenuous path are removed. The first gift of grace of the Master Maharshi, for example, is the widening (i.e., expansion) of the intuition of his devotee. Speaking practically, what is that intuition?

It is knowledge without thinking and action without forethought, all with the best possible results. Intuition may also come as a reward for well-performed practice in the study of the one-pointedness of the mind, and it will be in the form of genuine meditation, leading to the spiritual ecstasy of Samadhi.

If you reach the level of intuitional wisdom, then you will know that it comes, as does every spiritual boon, from the ability to establish inside of you a natural, tranquil *silence*. You will simply stop your thinking when you are in need of an especially important decision or action. Few would recognize this strange fact, aside from those who know about it beyond all doubt from their own experience.

And again I am compelled to stress the weight and necessity of a strict performance of the contents of Part III. For without it how can you maintain ten minutes of absolute freedom from all the intruders in your consciousness?

Perhaps some readers would like to use what has just been said about the powers of intuition, without passing through the unavoidable training. But in such a case only disappointment will be in store. I know of instances where people, having listened to what you have just read, tried to eject all thoughts when they needed to make an important decision or step. The result was usually worse than would have been achieved by simple, honest thinking out of the whole problem. Only emptiness was the answer, plus the time lost and the hope destroyed. Care is always needed, and not any expectation of getting *"something for nothing."*

One of the signs of advance along the path is the disappearance of our "I" of yesterday, when observed from today's point of view. It is the best proof of deep changes in a man. And we need a great deal of changing before we reach the unchangeable Reality within us.

But we should not allow any thought concerning the past to enter our consciousness, for it will inevitably destroy our concentration, which is dissipated by passionate retrospection. Later, after the advanced exercises have been duly performed and become your constant companions, a natural, wonderful tendency will arise in you. That is "to be without thought," to be in the *silence,* every moment the world's demands require no further tribute from you. In the presence of the master, this faculty, and many others, arise as if automatically, and the fruits of concentration can be reaped much earlier than otherwise.

The choice of the material for meditation—insofar as we have not yet arrived at the *mute* form of this wisdom—is very important. It must give us considerable service, though presented in however short a form. For that purpose, in the second English edition and in all translations of *In Days of Great Peace,* a special Appendix has been added at the end of the book. As stated previously, a large number of specially selected verses from the *Viveka-Chudamani* by Sankaracharya have been offered to the reader and student in a suitable sequence. From these inspired words, he can choose for himself the verses which evoke a particular response in him. He may use them in order to magnetize his mind and stimulate his intuition, in preparation for the highest form, leading to Samadhi. This finds its support in the following words of Sri Maharshi, speaking to his devotees: "To read Ribhu-Gita is as good as Samadhi."

Many inquiries occur when people hear about the state of consciousness of the future—the Samadhi. When we go upstairs, one foot cannot be raised from the lower step until the other has found secure support on the higher step. We cannot remain suspended in space. So, when we transfer the consciousness into the higher realm, we have to find some definite basis in the higher before we can leave the lower level. This is the answer to those who ask: "If there is another more real world, *why* cannot I see it in this one? If there is no death in that one, *why* do I have to die here?"

The aims and efforts of such people in this world have been concentrated solely on the physical life. How many try with the same effort of concentration to discover the Real, the goal of the Direct Path?

If we wish to achieve anything, we have first to make the effort. Is, then, the greatest of all possible achievements—the *resurrection from the deadly dream of matter*—to be gained cheaply? But there is always a small minority among men who are very different from their brothers. They are not too much concerned with the usual ways of life, having other aims to pursue.

These people are seeking quite a different kind of happiness from that of the average man. If they belong to a Western religion, their outer teachings have as a center God, more or less according to the dogmas involved.

If they are Easterners, their revelations may be different, often having a purely philosophical and abstract character. But with all of them, whether we call them saints or yogis, one thing in common can be observed. They live in another world, these men who find true bliss and the real purpose of their existence in a realm invisible and nonexistent for us.

The supreme test for a man—his death, or rather, the leaving of his physical form—holds no terror for these unique people. Spiritually awakened men do not consider physical destruction as the greatest evil that can befall a human being. Rather, for them it is liberation, a transition to the higher and more perfect life. The cardinal difference between these resurrected men and others lies in the state of their consciousness.

The former see things in another light and their reactions are unlike those of laymen. What makes the latter happy or unhappy has little or no influence on them. Certain of such men have given us messages of absolute authority, which could only come from a definite experience in the realm about which they speak. Sometimes these revelations have been of such power that many men already inwardly indifferent to worldly things have become "converted" and have followed the new path.

If we could ask them what happened, and why they so suddenly changed their ideas and strivings in life, their answer would often be: "Now I see everything from another point of view. What before was of overwhelming importance to me no longer has any meaning; for I see men and their activities, qualities, emotions, thoughts and fates, as from another world. The causes and effects are now much clearer to my inner sight and the inward dissonances and fears have disappeared forever."

And once again we see that it was just the state of consciousness which changed and nothing more. Nevertheless, we say that such a man became "quite another person."

What does it mean, that some of our brothers possess such a different and far wider state of consciousness, which others cannot even guess at?

The simplest and perhaps the most appropriate answer is that for the majority, the time has not yet come, for ripeness is a product of time in the life of the individual being, i.e., of those who still bear the burden of that most primitive form of self-consciousness in man—the *ego*. Although there cannot be any doubt that all men are brothers, since they belong to the same form of manifested life called humanity, *equality* does not, and never did, exist among them. However, we can be sure that in some future epoch mankind will reach a higher level of development. The forerunners, those few who are already nearing the goal, are a guarantee of that fact.

But we have said that man is *none* other than consciousness. Therefore, the sublime level of that consciousness, which we so much admire in a few highly developed men, is undoubtedly the heritage for future ages of humanity.

Different "initiations" are often spoken about; but after what we know from the foregoing chapters, we can conclude that *true initiation* can never be expressed in words. It simply means the *transformation of man,* and not certain secrets whispered in one's ear or written on paper. An analogy may be drawn to the idea of vaccination. Therefore, there cannot be false initiations, merely the *absence* of the true one.

But we might still be anxious to know, in our clumsy language of the mind, *what* is true initiation, or at least an approximate idea of it.

Knowing the impossibility of achieving exactness in this, it can merely be said that only true initiation gives knowledge of one's own being, and its relation to the Whole. This relation is invariably conceived of as union with the Whole.

The burning question for most seekers of spiritual attainment is how to enter on the path. We have some authoritative revelations on that matter from a contemporary master. Many already know theoretically what they have to do; sacred books of many old religions speak about the requisite qualities and there is no mystery about them.

There is not space here to enumerate the details and so only the outline will be recalled. It is: man must become harmless to everyone and everything; he must be good in his actions; and his intentions (or heart) should become pure.

The Maharshi added: "Now—accept in practice what you accept in theory." *That is the key to your resurrection into the new consciousness.*

We have already stated that the course of concentration should always be controlled once it has been successfully completed. That is because we began the whole operation of practical study with our still imperfect and unconquered mind, but finished with the elimination—or near elimination—of it as a compulsory factor in our conscious life (see exercises 8, 8A, 9 and 9A). Mind is like an ocean, which never remains in a state of absolute stillness. The only way to become free is to transcend that mind.

We learned to impose this stillness artificially, because of our ultimate separation from the thinking apparatus.

As a result, many new ways have been opened to us, because of our new abilities. Concentration was only the first real, although very important, step. It is something like matriculation, after which university training is open to us.

Now you can stop at this degree of attainment, satisfied with the results obtained, which will often put you far ahead of other men in your own class. You can develop your latent abilities to see things which no ordinary human eye can observe: i.e., the thoughts and feelings of another, by first concentrating your *active* attention on the person in question for a very short time, then immediately entering into the passive state of mind, in order to receive the *first* impressions coming from the other person's mind.

You can, by sharpening your will power through constant repetition of the advanced series of exercises (Chapters XVIII-XX), not only in secluded places but *under all possible conditions,* direct a single chosen thought into the mind you want to influence or test. The thought will be accepted and eventually you may master that mind, making it obedient to you.

If you use pranayama more extensively, prolonging the tempo of your breathing beyond your normal one, you may discover yet other possibilities of directing the pranic currents according to your will. First, of course, in your body, and then in those of others. Phenomena like mesmerism can be produced, and cures practiced if you are prepared to undertake additional study in a course of personal magnetism. For with the ability of concentration your field of activity may become very wide. If you have a friend who has also successfully performed this course, many telepathic experiences, and *these genuine ones,* can be conducted if you take turns being *transmitter and receiver.*

But if the *spirit of Sankaracharya,* still alive in you after Nos. 9 and 9A, *does attract you,* then things may have a much more serious implication. You may search for the rustless key, which will destroy the need for any more exercises, and which will lead you beyond this unreal world of changes and differences.

Then again remember the great inquiry—the Vichara—and substitute it for all exercises, thereby obtaining Wisdom instead of mere knowledge. There is nothing higher which spiritual teachers can offer to their disciples, providing the latter are able to accept it.

No visible reward is the lot of the successful adept of self-realization. In his outer aspects he apparently remains what he was before, as the Direct Path is a *secret* one.

You will never be entitled to tell the world that you have reached your goal. Briefly, there will be no one left in you who could utter anything like that. Your ego-personality will have died long ago, and you—the Self, silent, omnipresent, omniscient—cannot speak of such things to the shadows of the dream world.

Long before your enlightenment you will enter into constant communion with the present master of that sublime path. He will direct your steps and supervise—from inside yourself— your real growth. If you want to anticipate what a communion with the master, whom you never met in this physical life, *is,* then read another book, written by a man who, after a life rich in experiences, hopes, blunders, but always filled with the indomitable spirit of search for the Truth of life, finally found his guru, destined for him by Providence.

This book is entitled *Initiations* by Paul Sédir of Paris. From it you will learn how the impossible becomes possible, and how things happen which are the true cause of human history, but about which men know so little.

On the Direct Path the process of acquiring virtues is reversed. One does not seek them, for they come of themselves according to the measure of your advancement along the thorny path. To compel ourselves to seek virtues is practically as useless as to fly from temptations.

We all know that no true victory can be won by flight, only by vigorous and courageous fighting. And we must know what we are fighting against, otherwise we will be on the losing side. It is only the Direct Path which tells us, from the first step, *where* we are going and—*why.*

Our renunciation of this unreal world, while *usually not known or perceptible to those around us,* acquires *a natural* and *reasonable* character, and not that of imagination or hazy dreams. Then we experientially know the true value of the things belonging to the world of senses, in the midst of which we are still living, in our physical shells.

I realize that many people must apparently still follow the doubtful ways, for they are unable to appreciate the *only way,* which leads to the ultimate achievement. And in that sense we can accept—to a certain degree—that "all paths lead to the same goal," for "time itself is flowing away into eternity."

The Direct Path also agrees with the spiritual testament of the Lord Buddha himself: "You cannot destroy your illusions by creating other illusions in their place."

Have you not yet realized the wonderful condition which forms the title and subject of this final chapter? Reading, writing, walking—have you never had some moments when you were apart from your personality, merged in the untroubled, all-penetrating peace, in which there are no contradictions, desires, inquiries and other attributes of the lower state of consciousness, so common to all our fellow men? Has this not happened to you, after you practiced exercise No. 9A for some time, which was inspired by the spirit of Sankara? If not, then know that it is quite possible to write, speak and perform many other worldly activities, and at the same time to be "out of this world."

The condition for this is natural simplicity and lack of all unnecessary, complicated and compulsory thinking and striving in you. I hope that by now you may have guessed that this comes as a result of the control of one's mind. And, I repeat, that control is nothing else than the ability and the bliss of inducing the state of inner stillness, from which you can look down on everything with an eye of wisdom, and not with the eyes of the world troubled by passions and their parents—ignorance and shallowness of consciousness. All these things are the signs of the Resurrection.

When I try to transfer that term into the current language, so that you may read and get from it some mental approach to the idea which has dictated these lines, *serenity* and *seriousness* are the only aspects of the experience which can be translated. In the thoughtless world, in which life is no longer veiled by the shrouds of matter, the fact of resurrection, when it happens to the person concerned, is beyond all doubt. It means that the former troublesome states of the three-plane life are seen to be nonlife, a parody and an unworthy substitute for life.

This does not create morbid or negative currents in a man. For the fact of *knowing* what has been said in the foregoing sentence is not connected with suffering or resentment. These things do not exist in the realm of the permanent light.

The one expression which has perhaps more affinity with human language, the consequence of the fourth state after our resurrection in spirit, might be the conception of freedom. It is *absolute freedom,* and only one who has succeeded in winning the battle with the arch-troublemaker—mind—can appreciate this aspect of realization.

We really remain enslaved by this life until we win that battle, in which the main weapon is concentration. Only then can we enjoy independence from everything which binds us in the world of relativity.

When the student looks back on the course of concentration he has just completed, he will see that the experiences were of the kind which exclude, one after another, all the senses of the physical body, without resulting in the state of sleep or swoon.

Let us make a final analysis in summarized form.

First and Second Series:

Exercises Nos. 1, 1A and 2 and 2A exclude your sight and hearing. The A and B of Chapter XVII let you understand some useful manifestations of the magnetic forces and their currents in nature, from their invisible sources in the sun and moon.

Third Series:

Exercises Nos. 3 and 3A develop a peculiar kind of sight, which extends itself beyond our three physical dimensions.

Nos. (*a*) and (*b*) of Chapter XVIII teach us to use the means of active defense against incoming thoughts and emotions.

Fourth Series:

Nos. 4 and 4A develop actively intense concentration using the powers of visualization.

Nos. 5 and 5A develop a flexible imagination about chosen

objects, the concentration acting as a strong background as in all the former exercises.

Nos. 6 and 6A develop passive concentration, beyond sight and hearing.

Fifth Series:

Exercises Nos. 7 and 7A deal with a combination of the active and passive forms.

And the two final groups of Nos. 8 and 8A and 9 and 9A develop the highest degree of the passive form and that of the expansion of the mind to the very point where we are able to transcend it, thereby losing all contact with visible and tangible manifestations.

The term "spiritual master" has been frequently mentioned throughout this book, and it seems to me that some explanation should be given before closing this last chapter. Some will prefer to stop their study with the completion of the exercises up to Nos. 8 and 8A and use the abilities so gained for their everyday life. They are perfectly free to do so. But some will try to go further and to extend their search, armed with concentration, to the nonmaterial realm. For such students, more information about the spiritual guides, i.e., the true masters, may be of *great* value.

If the finding of a master is an essential condition for all spiritual attainment, then questions like the two that follow may arise. How can this be accomplished? And how can we recognize the master and so avoid any errors in our quest? Such questions are perfectly natural and can and should be answered.

Properly speaking, the key to the finding and recognition of a true master (Sad-Guru) lies within each one of us. In ordinary language, the best definition of such a master would be—an ideal man. Nothing short of that can really attract the eternal element in the prospective disciple and hold him until the glorious end is reached. As can readily be seen, such men cannot be numerous or easily found. In fact, humanity records only a few of these great personages in all its history. But there have been, and still are, many minor saints and yogis, as well as unsuccessful disciples of a genuine master, who wish to present themselves as true masters.

No matter how good and sincere their intentions may be, the very fact of their striving to appear what they are not speaks for itself. Discrimination and keen insight should be two of the cardinal virtues of every disciple about to embark upon the path to inner progress.

Christ warned us when he said: "For many shall come in my name, saying, I am Christ; and shall deceive many."

The spiritual master of the present epoch repeated the same warning, pointing out clearly that the so-called "ordinary saints and yogis" are only slightly more advanced men, whose powers are still limited and who are not as yet free from the deadly "primordial sin" which is ignorance. Even in everyday life, a person only partially trained in teaching would not be engaged as a schoolmaster because he would be unable to prove full professional ability.

In the spiritual realm, such a leader, who is himself not yet free from all human weaknesses and ignorance, cannot possibly answer the human longing for the sublime ideal, which should be satisfied. Moreover, he can easily mislead those who lack the necessary discriminatory power and who consequently might wrongly attach themselves to a false teacher.

Now we shall examine the qualities of a true master of wisdom who has a real message for suffering mankind:

a. The master invariably comes into this world ripe, and endowed with all spiritual perfection, which manifests as soon as his childhood is over and early manhood begins. The true master does not spend the first part of his earthly life leading an average human existence, i.e., committing the common sins, and then only in the second part becoming "converted" and living as a saint or yogi. Any person who does so, who, after recognition of the true teacher, forsakes the wrong path, may well become a successful disciple. He will still have plenty of work ahead of him. His karma is far from finished and he will still have to pay an enormous number of "debts," while on the other hand a true guru or Jivanmukta is forever free. We may honor such advanced students of the great school of life, but we should never dare to compare them to a perfect being, a Sad-Guru, who is without any blemish, with no past, present or future, and who is without the slightest trace of "ego."

b. The guru has no attachments. He is not affected by, or interested in, the number of his adherents (devotees), for he knows that whoever is mature enough will eventually find his way to the master even from the farthermost corner of the earth. Therefore, there is no need for a Sad-Guru to travel in order to propagate his teachings. Such behavior would be inconsistent and incompatible with the greatness and wisdom of a perfect man.

c. The true master is far beyond and above all existing religions, although he does not condemn any of them, knowing that they are the first necessary steps for less advanced human beings. Consequently he does not favor any particular creed and is not concerned with the so-called "conversions" or changes of religion.

d. The guru leads an exemplary and perfectly unattached life, showing us how we can transcend all our limitations which so often seem insurmountable. Like a beacon, he sheds, in all directions, the light of his example, of his attainment, and his unity with the cosmic Self-God.

e. He refuses to possess anything in this material world. Therefore, he gives the lie to the old saying, which allegedly states that no one can live without attachment to earthly things.

f. He has no personal relationships in our sense of the word. He is beyond all ties of family or society. At the same time, those who find such a master acquire a true and great friend, to whom everyone can turn for help and inspiration.

g. No true master talks or writes very much. Sometimes, like Christ or Buddha he does not write at all, or like the Maharshi very little. Why? Because he knows that some of his directly inspired disciples will invariably perform all the needed technical work in order to transmit his message to humanity. This leaves him more time and freedom for higher, purely spiritual, constructive and invisible work in this world. The master never argues with anyone.

h. He does not accept any gifts and condescends to take only a little of the things his body needs. All other attitudes adopted by those who like to pose as "masters" are at best only self-deception or they may simply be deceiving others. For, in our time, we have legions of such false and therefore highly dangerous "masters," who are ready to "help" or "initiate" us, providing we can afford to pay them. Only utterly blind or decadent people could accept such "guidance" for which they have to pay in money or some other form of material goods.

i. The true masters do not usually exhibit siddhis (occult powers) for they transcended them long ago when they were still on the threshold of masterhood. A true master possesses all siddhis and infinitely more for he is *one* with the unmanifested Supreme, which is the source of all power.

j. No Jivanmukta accepts any pet names, superfluous titles or other symbols of human emotions. It would be too far below his dignity and wisdom. The great rishi of our own epoch told us that, "in truth, he does not possess any name at all." For a name given by men means personality, ego or a label. While a genuine teacher has left his former "ego" in the far-off past, numerous self-styled "masters" of today still like pompous and empty titles as well as cheap adoration from undiscriminating people. Their egos are still strong and far from extinct.

k. The master is utterly indifferent to his physical existence, his body being only a shell, although perhaps of importance to us, his devotees, who are still accustomed to look first on material forms. But this body is without any meaning to the illimitable spiritual consciousness of a true master. He is not eager to dispose of the body before the proper time, nor would he make any effort to retain it when it is dying. Only ordinary men run to doctors for medicines. Shortly before leaving the physical form, the great Rishi Ramana said: "This body *itself* is a disease!" That is an initiation and the ultimate truth about this physical existence which is so much cherished by ignorant people. The sage knows that everything happens in due course, so how could he oppose what is inevitable?

l. Only the perfect man can teach in silence, because he has reached it, and therefore he alone can stimulate it in others. He speaks through the silence infinitely more potently than through any human language. But those who are not yet Jivanmuktas naturally prefer to use speech and pen.

m. Another sign for recognition of a true master who has a spiritual message for humanity is the fact that he never has any earthly master himself. He comes ripe and ready to open for us new spiritual paths and needs no human help. Such was the case with Christ, Buddha and Ramana Maharshi; but lesser leaders have helpers similar to themselves. Therefore, let us associate ourselves with the foremost.

These are only a few points, but nevertheless they may help many sincere seekers and students to escape from the otherwise unavoidable and bitter disappointments which ensue if they do not follow a genuine master. If their power of discrimination is not strong enough, they may accept only a shadow substitute instead of a true guru. You can imagine the immense harm which might result from such a mistake.

We should realize that a true spiritual master, who has a

definite mission in this world, is beyond all conditions and is unaffected by the surrounding average people. His power is too great to allow our impure and disorderly vibrations, which we undoubtedly emit because of our imperfections—passions and foolishness—to disturb his eternal peace of unity with the Absolute Whole. Such a master (Christ, Buddha, Maharshi) does not hide himself in inaccessible places, but performs his work amongst us without any grievance or difficulty. Those who act differently are not true and perfect masters. If we wish to tread the thorny path of perfection and liberation— the *Direct Path,* which is the only one that can give immediate results to spiritually mature people—then we should consider only the one who has a message for his own epoch.

Such a path has just been opened for us by the great rishi. And a few saints and devotees who have only partially accepted the gist of the rishi's message have since tried to found schools in their own names and based on their "own" teachings.

Some may object that such a high standard for a guru, as stated above, does not really exist and has not yet been reached by any human being. *That is absolutely wrong.* For there are still many living men who saw such a master, listened to his words and perceived spiritual horizons which were opened for them by his light. This shortened their experiences and immensely helped them toward spiritual awakening. They know that the master possesses much more than has been mentioned. Also, we know that he passed away physically only a few years ago.

That is why all sincere devotees of a true guru *refuse to accept any other guidance* or to submit to any of the numerous self-styled "masters" who are so easily accepted by many other people. To them, the communion with the Sad-Guru means all for which they can wish and toil. One who has abandoned untruth for Truth cannot reverse the process any more than a river can retrieve its waters from the ocean. The taste of the eternal, reached by contact with the true guru, means everything to many of us.

There is not much left to say now apart from extending the author's sincerest wishes for success to all earnest students. If this book has helped some people to raise their inner standard to a higher one, that would be the best reward for both writer and student alike. Wandering through this earthly life, we may often forget to inquire properly into the aim of that wandering. So as an epilogue let us meditate on a beautiful excerpt from the ancient Upanishads:

> As the eagle of the mountains, having soared high in the air above the earth,
> Wings its way back to its resting place, being fatigued by its long flight,
> So does the soul, having experienced the life of the phenomenal, relative and mortal,
> Return finally unto itself, where it can sleep beyond all desires, and beyond all dreams. . . .

MELVIN POWERS SELF-IMPROVEMENT LIBRARY

ASTROLOGY

____ ASTROLOGY: HOW TO CHART YOUR HOROSCOPE *Max Heindel*	5.00
____ ASTROLOGY AND SEXUAL ANALYSIS *Morris C. Goodman*	5.00
____ ASTROLOGY AND YOU *Carroll Righter*	5.00
____ ASTROLOGY MADE EASY *Astarte*	5.00
____ ASTROLOGY, ROMANCE, YOU AND THE STARS *Anthony Norvell*	5.00
____ MY WORLD OF ASTROLOGY *Sydney Omarr*	7.00
____ THOUGHT DIAL *Sydney Omarr*	7.00
____ WHAT THE STARS REVEAL ABOUT THE MEN IN YOUR LIFE *Thelma White*	3.00

BRIDGE

____ BRIDGE BIDDING MADE EASY *Edwin B. Kantar*	10.00
____ BRIDGE CONVENTIONS *Edwin B. Kantar*	10.00
____ COMPETITIVE BIDDING IN MODERN BRIDGE *Edgar Kaplan*	7.00
____ DEFENSIVE BRIDGE PLAY COMPLETE *Edwin B. Kantar*	15.00
____ GAMESMAN BRIDGE–PLAY BETTER WITH KANTAR *Edwin B. Kantar*	7.00
____ HOW TO IMPROVE YOUR BRIDGE *Alfred Sheinwold*	7.00
____ IMPROVING YOUR BIDDING SKILLS *Edwin B. Kantar*	7.00
____ INTRODUCTION TO DECLARER'S PLAY *Edwin B. Kantar*	7.00
____ INTRODUCTION TO DEFENDER'S PLAY *Edwin B. Kantar*	7.00
____ KANTAR FOR THE DEFENSE *Edwin B. Kantar*	7.00
____ KANTAR FOR THE DEFENSE VOLUME 2 *Edwin B. Kantar*	7.00
____ TEST YOUR BRIDGE PLAY *Edwin B. Kantar*	7.00
____ VOLUME 2–TEST YOUR BRIDGE PLAY *Edwin B. Kantar*	7.00
____ WINNING DECLARER PLAY *Dorothy Hayden Truscott*	7.00

BUSINESS, STUDY & REFERENCE

____ BRAINSTORMING *Charles Clark*	7.00
____ CONVERSATION MADE EASY *Elliot Russell*	5.00
____ EXAM SECRET *Dennis B. Jackson*	5.00
____ FIX-IT BOOK *Arthur Symons*	2.00
____ HOW TO DEVELOP A BETTER SPEAKING VOICE *M. Hellier*	4.00
____ HOW TO SAVE 50% ON GAS & CAR EXPENSES *Ken Stansbie*	5.00
____ HOW TO SELF-PUBLISH YOUR BOOK & MAKE IT A BEST SELLER *Melvin Powers*	20.00
____ INCREASE YOUR LEARNING POWER *Geoffrey A. Dudley*	3.00
____ PRACTICAL GUIDE TO BETTER CONCENTRATION *Melvin Powers*	5.00
____ 7 DAYS TO FASTER READING *William S. Schaill*	7.00
____ SONGWRITERS' RHYMING DICTIONARY *Jane Shaw Whitfield*	10.00
____ SPELLING MADE EASY *Lester D. Basch & Dr. Milton Finkelstein*	3.00
____ STUDENT'S GUIDE TO BETTER GRADES *J. A. Rickard*	3.00
____ TEST YOURSELF–FIND YOUR HIDDEN TALENT *Jack Shafer*	3.00
____ YOUR WILL & WHAT TO DO ABOUT IT *Attorney Samuel G. Kling*	5.00

CALLIGRAPHY

____ ADVANCED CALLIGRAPHY *Katherine Jeffares*	7.00
____ CALLIGRAPHY–THE ART OF BEAUTIFUL WRITING *Katherine Jeffares*	7.00
____ CALLIGRAPHY FOR FUN & PROFIT *Anne Leptich & Jacque Evans*	7.00
____ CALLIGRAPHY MADE EASY *Tina Serafini*	7.00

CHESS & CHECKERS

____ BEGINNER'S GUIDE TO WINNING CHESS *Fred Reinfeld*	5.00
____ CHESS IN TEN EASY LESSONS *Larry Evans*	5.00
____ CHESS MADE EASY *Milton L. Hanauer*	5.00
____ CHESS PROBLEMS FOR BEGINNERS *Edited by Fred Reinfeld*	5.00
____ CHESS TACTICS FOR BEGINNERS *Edited by Fred Reinfeld*	5.00

_____ HOW TO WIN AT CHECKERS *Fred Reinfeld*   5.00
_____ 1001 BRILLIANT WAYS TO CHECKMATE *Fred Reinfeld*   7.00
_____ 1001 WINNING CHESS SACRIFICES & COMBINATIONS *Fred Reinfeld*   7.00

COOKERY & HERBS
_____ CULPEPER'S HERBAL REMEDIES *Dr. Nicholas Culpeper*   5.00
_____ FAST GOURMET COOKBOOK *Poppy Cannon*   2.50
_____ HEALING POWER OF HERBS *May Bethel*   5.00
_____ HEALING POWER OF NATURAL FOODS *May Bethel*   5.00
_____ HERBS FOR HEALTH—HOW TO GROW & USE THEM *Louise Evans Doole*   5.00
_____ HOME GARDEN COOKBOOK—DELICIOUS NATURAL FOOD RECIPES *Ken Kraft*   3.00
_____ MEATLESS MEAL GUIDE *Tomi Ryan & James H. Ryan, M.D.*   4.00
_____ VEGETABLE GARDENING FOR BEGINNERS *Hugh Wiberg*   2.00
_____ VEGETABLES FOR TODAY'S GARDENS *R. Milton Carleton*   2.00
_____ VEGETARIAN COOKERY *Janet Walker*   7.00
_____ VEGETARIAN COOKING MADE EASY & DELECTABLE *Veronica Vezza*   3.00
_____ VEGETARIAN DELIGHTS—A HAPPY COOKBOOK FOR HEALTH *K. R. Mehta*   2.00
_____ VEGETARIAN GOURMET COOKBOOK *Joyce McKinnel*   3.00

GAMBLING & POKER
_____ HOW TO WIN AT DICE GAMES *Skip Frey*   3.00
_____ HOW TO WIN AT POKER *Terence Reese & Anthony T. Watkins*   7.00
_____ SCARNE ON DICE *John Scarne*   15.00
_____ WINNING AT CRAPS *Dr. Lloyd T. Commins*   5.00
_____ WINNING AT GIN *Chester Wander & Cy Rice*   3.00
_____ WINNING AT POKER—AN EXPERT'S GUIDE *John Archer*   5.00
_____ WINNING AT 21—AN EXPERT'S GUIDE *John Archer*   7.00
_____ WINNING POKER SYSTEMS *Norman Zadeh*   3.00

HEALTH
_____ BEE POLLEN *Lynda Lyngheim & Jack Scagnetti*   3.00
_____ COPING WITH ALZHEIMER'S *Rose Oliver, Ph.D. & Francis Bock, Ph.D.*   10.00
_____ DR. LINDNER'S POINT SYSTEM FOOD PROGRAM *Peter G. Lindner, M.D.*   2.00
_____ HELP YOURSELF TO BETTER SIGHT *Margaret Darst Corbett*   7.00
_____ HOW YOU CAN STOP SMOKING PERMANENTLY *Ernest Caldwell*   5.00
_____ MIND OVER PLATTER *Peter G. Lindner, M.D.*   5.00
_____ NATURE'S WAY TO NUTRITION & VIBRANT HEALTH *Robert J. Scrutton*   3.00
_____ NEW CARBOHYDRATE DIET COUNTER *Patti Lopez-Pereira*   2.00
_____ REFLEXOLOGY *Dr. Maybelle Segal*   5.00
_____ REFLEXOLOGY FOR GOOD HEALTH *Anna Kaye & Don C. Matchan*   7.00
_____ 30 DAYS TO BEAUTIFUL LEGS *Dr. Marc Selner*   3.00
_____ YOU CAN LEARN TO RELAX *Dr. Samuel Gutwirth*   3.00

HOBBIES
_____ BEACHCOMBING FOR BEGINNERS *Norman Hickin*   2.00
_____ BLACKSTONE'S MODERN CARD TRICKS *Harry Blackstone*   5.00
_____ BLACKSTONE'S SECRETS OF MAGIC *Harry Blackstone*   5.00
_____ COIN COLLECTING FOR BEGINNERS *Burton Hobson & Fred Reinfeld*   7.00
_____ ENTERTAINING WITH ESP *Tony 'Doc' Shiels*   2.00
_____ 400 FASCINATING MAGIC TRICKS YOU CAN DO *Howard Thurston*   7.00
_____ HOW I TURN JUNK INTO FUN AND PROFIT *Sari*   3.00
_____ HOW TO WRITE A HIT SONG & SELL IT *Tommy Boyce*   7.00
_____ MAGIC FOR ALL AGES *Walter Gibson*   4.00
_____ STAMP COLLECTING FOR BEGINNERS *Burton Hobson*   3.00

HORSE PLAYER'S WINNING GUIDES
_____ BETTING HORSES TO WIN *Les Conklin*   7.00
_____ ELIMINATE THE LOSERS *Bob McKnight*   5.00
_____ HOW TO PICK WINNING HORSES *Bob McKnight*   5.00

___ HOW TO WIN AT THE RACES *Sam (The Genius) Lewin*	5.00
___ HOW YOU CAN BEAT THE RACES *Jack Kavanaqh*	5.00
___ MAKING MONEY AT THE RACES *David Barr*	5.00
___ PAYDAY AT THE RACES *Les Conklin*	5.00
___ SMART HANDICAPPING MADE EASY *William Bauman*	5.00
___ SUCCESS AT THE HARNESS RACES *Barry Meadow*	5.00

HUMOR

___ HOW TO FLATTEN YOUR TUSH *Coach Marge Reardon*	2.00
___ HOW TO MAKE LOVE TO YOURSELF *Ron Stevens & Joy Grdnic*	3.00
___ JOKE TELLER'S HANDBOOK *Bob Orben*	7.00
___ JOKES FOR ALL OCCASIONS *Al Schock*	5.00
___ 2,000 NEW LAUGHS FOR SPEAKERS *Bob Orben*	7.00
___ 2,400 JOKES TO BRIGHTEN YOUR SPEECHES *Robert Orben*	7.00
___ 2,500 JOKES TO START 'EM LAUGHING *Bob Orben*	7.00

HYPNOTISM

___ ADVANCED TECHNIQUES OF HYPNOSIS *Melvin Powers*	3.00
___ CHILDBIRTH WITH HYPNOSIS *William S. Kroger, M.D.*	5.00
___ HOW TO SOLVE YOUR SEX PROBLEMS WITH SELF-HYPNOSIS *Frank S. Caprio, M.D.*	5.00
___ HOW TO STOP SMOKING THRU SELF-HYPNOSIS *Leslie M. LeCron*	3.00
___ HOW YOU CAN BOWL BETTER USING SELF-HYPNOSIS *Jack Heise*	4.00
___ HOW YOU CAN PLAY BETTER GOLF USING SELF-HYPNOSIS *Jack Heise*	3.00
___ HYPNOSIS AND SELF-HYPNOSIS *Bernard Hollander, M.D.*	5.00
___ HYPNOTISM *(Originally published in 1893) Carl Sextus*	5.00
___ HYPNOTISM MADE EASY *Dr. Ralph Winn*	5.00
___ HYPNOTISM MADE PRACTICAL *Louis Orton*	5.00
___ HYPNOTISM REVEALED *Melvin Powers*	3.00
___ HYPNOTISM TODAY *Leslie LeCron and Jean Bordeaux, Ph.D.*	5.00
___ MODERN HYPNOSIS *Lesley Kuhn & Salvatore Russo, Ph.D.*	5.00
___ NEW CONCEPTS OF HYPNOSIS *Bernard C. Gindes, M.D.*	10.00
___ NEW SELF-HYPNOSIS *Paul Adams*	7.00
___ POST-HYPNOTIC INSTRUCTIONS—SUGGESTIONS FOR THERAPY *Arnold Furst*	5.00
___ PRACTICAL GUIDE TO SELF-HYPNOSIS *Melvin Powers*	5.00
___ PRACTICAL HYPNOTISM *Philip Magonet, M.D.*	3.00
___ SECRETS OF HYPNOTISM *S. J. Van Pelt, M.D.*	5.00
___ SELF-HYPNOSIS—A CONDITIONED-RESPONSE TECHNIQUE *Laurence Sparks*	7.00
___ SELF-HYPNOSIS—ITS THEORY, TECHNIQUE & APPLICATION *Melvin Powers*	3.00
___ THERAPY THROUGH HYPNOSIS *Edited by Raphael H. Rhodes*	5.00

JUDAICA

___ SERVICE OF THE HEART *Evelyn Garfiel, Ph.D.*	10.00
___ STORY OF ISRAEL IN COINS *Jean & Maurice Gould*	2.00
___ STORY OF ISRAEL IN STAMPS *Maxim & Gabriel Shamir*	1.00
___ TONGUE OF THE PROPHETS *Robert St. John*	7.00

JUST FOR WOMEN

___ COSMOPOLITAN'S GUIDE TO MARVELOUS MEN Foreword by *Helen Gurley Brown*	3.00
___ COSMOPOLITAN'S HANG-UP HANDBOOK Foreword by *Helen Gurley Brown*	4.00
___ COSMOPOLITAN'S LOVE BOOK—A GUIDE TO ECSTASY IN BED	7.00
___ COSMOPOLITAN'S NEW ETIQUETTE GUIDE Foreword by *Helen Gurley Brown*	4.00
___ I AM A COMPLEAT WOMAN *Doris Hagopian & Karen O'Connor Sweeney*	3.00
___ JUST FOR WOMEN—A GUIDE TO THE FEMALE BODY *Richard E. Sand, M.D.*	5.00
___ NEW APPROACHES TO SEX IN MARRIAGE *John E. Eichenlaub, M.D.*	3.00
___ SEXUALLY ADEQUATE FEMALE *Frank S. Caprio, M.D.*	3.00
___ SEXUALLY FULFILLED WOMAN *Dr. Rachel Copelan*	5.00

MARRIAGE, SEX & PARENTHOOD

___ ABILITY TO LOVE *Dr. Allan Fromme*	7.00
___ GUIDE TO SUCCESSFUL MARRIAGE *Drs. Albert Ellis & Robert Harper*	7.00
___ HOW TO RAISE AN EMOTIONALLY HEALTHY, HAPPY CHILD *Albert Ellis, Ph.D.*	7.00
___ PARENT SURVIVAL TRAINING *Marvin Silverman, Ed.D. & David Lustig, Ph.D.*	10.00
___ SEX WITHOUT GUILT *Albert Ellis, Ph.D.*	5.00
___ SEXUALLY ADEQUATE MALE *Frank S. Caprio, M.D.*	3.00
___ SEXUALLY FULFILLED MAN *Dr. Rachel Copelan*	5.00
___ STAYING IN LOVE *Dr. Norton F. Kristy*	7.00

MELVIN POWERS' MAIL ORDER LIBRARY

___ HOW TO GET RICH IN MAIL ORDER *Melvin Powers*	20.00
___ HOW TO SELF-PUBLISH YOUR BOOK & MAKE IT A BEST SELLER *Melvin Powers*	20.00
___ HOW TO WRITE A GOOD ADVERTISEMENT *Victor O. Schwab*	20.00
___ MAIL ORDER MADE EASY *J. Frank Brumbaugh*	20.00

METAPHYSICS & OCCULT

___ CONCENTRATION—A GUIDE TO MENTAL MASTERY *Mouni Sadhu*	7.00
___ EXTRA-TERRESTRIAL INTELLIGENCE—THE FIRST ENCOUNTER	6.00
___ FORTUNE TELLING WITH CARDS *P. Foli*	5.00
___ HOW TO INTERPRET DREAMS, OMENS & FORTUNE TELLING SIGNS *Gettings*	5.00
___ HOW TO UNDERSTAND YOUR DREAMS *Geoffrey A. Dudley*	5.00
___ IN DAYS OF GREAT PEACE *Mouni Sadhu*	3.00
___ MAGICIAN—HIS TRAINING AND WORK *W. E. Butler*	5.00
___ MEDITATION *Mouni Sadhu*	10.00
___ MODERN NUMEROLOGY *Morris C. Goodman*	5.00
___ NUMEROLOGY—ITS FACTS AND SECRETS *Ariel Yvon Taylor*	5.00
___ NUMEROLOGY MADE EASY *W. Mykian*	5.00
___ PALMISTRY MADE EASY *Fred Gettings*	5.00
___ PALMISTRY MADE PRACTICAL *Elizabeth Daniels Squire*	7.00
___ PALMISTRY SECRETS REVEALED *Henry Frith*	4.00
___ PROPHECY IN OUR TIME *Martin Ebon*	2.50
___ SUPERSTITION—ARE YOU SUPERSTITIOUS? *Eric Maple*	2.00
___ TAROT *Mouni Sadhu*	10.00
___ TAROT OF THE BOHEMIANS *Papus*	7.00
___ WAYS TO SELF-REALIZATION *Mouni Sadhu*	7.00
___ WITCHCRAFT, MAGIC & OCCULTISM—A FASCINATING HISTORY *W. B. Crow*	7.00
___ WITCHCRAFT—THE SIXTH SENSE *Justine Glass*	7.00

RECOVERY

___ KNIGHT IN RUSTY ARMOR *Robert Fisher*	5.00
___ KNIGHT IN RUSTY ARMOR *Robert Fisher (Hard cover edition)*	10.00

SELF-HELP & INSPIRATIONAL

___ CHARISMA—HOW TO GET "THAT SPECIAL MAGIC" *Marcia Grad*	7.00
___ DAILY POWER FOR JOYFUL LIVING *Dr. Donald Curtis*	7.00
___ DYNAMIC THINKING *Melvin Powers*	5.00
___ GREATEST POWER IN THE UNIVERSE *U. S. Andersen*	7.00
___ GROW RICH WHILE YOU SLEEP *Ben Sweetland*	7.00
___ GROW RICH WITH YOUR MILLION DOLLAR MIND *Brian Adams*	7.00
___ GROWTH THROUGH REASON *Albert Ellis, Ph.D.*	7.00
___ GUIDE TO PERSONAL HAPPINESS *Albert Ellis, Ph.D. & Irving Becker, Ed.D.*	7.00
___ HANDWRITING ANALYSIS MADE EASY *John Marley*	7.00
___ HANDWRITING TELLS *Nadya Olyanova*	7.00
___ HOW TO ATTRACT GOOD LUCK *A.H.Z. Carr*	7.00
___ HOW TO DEVELOP A WINNING PERSONALITY *Martin Panzer*	7.00
___ HOW TO DEVELOP AN EXCEPTIONAL MEMORY *Young & Gibson*	7.00
___ HOW TO LIVE WITH A NEUROTIC *Albert Ellis, Ph.D.*	7.00
___ HOW TO OVERCOME YOUR FEARS *M. P. Leahy, M.D.*	3.00
___ HOW TO SUCCEED *Brian Adams*	7.00

___ HUMAN PROBLEMS & HOW TO SOLVE THEM *Dr. Donald Curtis*	5.00
___ I CAN *Ben Sweetland*	8.00
___ I WILL *Ben Sweetland*	7.00
___ KNIGHT IN RUSTY ARMOR *Robert Fisher*	5.00
___ KNIGHT IN RUSTY ARMOR *Robert Fisher (Hard cover edition)*	10.00
___ LEFT-HANDED PEOPLE *Michael Barsley*	5.00
___ MAGIC IN YOUR MIND *U.S. Andersen*	10.00
___ MAGIC OF THINKING SUCCESS *Dr. David J. Schwartz*	7.00
___ MAGIC POWER OF YOUR MIND *Walter M. Germain*	7.00
___ MENTAL POWER THROUGH SLEEP SUGGESTION *Melvin Powers*	3.00
___ NEVER UNDERESTIMATE THE SELLING POWER OF A WOMAN *Dottie Walters*	7.00
___ NEW GUIDE TO RATIONAL LIVING *Albert Ellis, Ph.D. & R. Harper, Ph.D.*	7.00
___ PSYCHO-CYBERNETICS *Maxwell Maltz, M.D.*	7.00
___ PSYCHOLOGY OF HANDWRITING *Nadya Olyanova*	7.00
___ SALES CYBERNETICS *Brian Adams*	10.00
___ SCIENCE OF MIND IN DAILY LIVING *Dr. Donald Curtis*	7.00
___ SECRET OF SECRETS *U.S. Andersen*	7.00
___ SECRET POWER OF THE PYRAMIDS *U. S. Andersen*	7.00
___ SELF-THERAPY FOR THE STUTTERER *Malcolm Frazer*	3.00
___ SUCCESS-CYBERNETICS *U. S. Andersen*	7.00
___ 10 DAYS TO A GREAT NEW LIFE *William E. Edwards*	3.00
___ THINK AND GROW RICH *Napoleon Hill*	8.00
___ THREE MAGIC WORDS *U. S. Andersen*	7.00
___ TREASURY OF COMFORT *Edited by Rabbi Sidney Greenberg*	10.00
___ TREASURY OF THE ART OF LIVING *Sidney S. Greenberg*	7.00
___ WHAT YOUR HANDWRITING REVEALS *Albert E. Hughes*	4.00
___ YOUR SUBCONSCIOUS POWER *Charles M. Simmons*	7.00
___ YOUR THOUGHTS CAN CHANGE YOUR LIFE *Dr. Donald Curtis*	7.00

SPORTS

___ BILLIARDS—POCKET • CAROM • THREE CUSHION *Clive Cottingham, Jr.*	5.00
___ COMPLETE GUIDE TO FISHING *Vlad Evanoff*	2.00
___ HOW TO IMPROVE YOUR RACQUETBALL *Lubarsky, Kaufman & Scagnetti*	5.00
___ HOW TO WIN AT POCKET BILLIARDS *Edward D. Knuchell*	7.00
___ JOY OF WALKING *Jack Scagnetti*	3.00
___ LEARNING & TEACHING SOCCER SKILLS *Eric Worthington*	3.00
___ MOTORCYCLING FOR BEGINNERS *I.G. Edmonds*	3.00
___ RACQUETBALL FOR WOMEN *Toni Hudson, Jack Scagnetti & Vince Rondone*	3.00
___ RACQUETBALL MADE EASY *Steve Lubarsky, Rod Delson & Jack Scagnetti*	5.00
___ SECRET OF BOWLING STRIKES *Dawson Taylor*	5.00
___ SOCCER—THE GAME & HOW TO PLAY IT *Gary Rosenthal*	7.00
___ STARTING SOCCER *Edward F. Dolan, Jr.*	3.00

TENNIS LOVER'S LIBRARY

___ HOW TO BEAT BETTER TENNIS PLAYERS *Loring Fiske*	4.00
___ PSYCH YOURSELF TO BETTER TENNIS *Dr. Walter A. Luszki*	2.00
___ TENNIS FOR BEGINNERS *Dr. H. A. Murray*	2.00
___ TENNIS MADE EASY *Joel Brecheen*	5.00
___ WEEKEND TENNIS—HOW TO HAVE FUN & WIN AT THE SAME TIME *Bill Talbert*	3.00

WILSHIRE PET LIBRARY

___ DOG TRAINING MADE EASY & FUN *John W. Kellogg*	5.00
___ HOW TO BRING UP YOUR PET DOG *Kurt Unkelbach*	2.00
___ HOW TO RAISE & TRAIN YOUR PUPPY *Jeff Griffen*	5.00

The books listed above can be obtained from your book dealer or directly from Melvin Powers.
When ordering, please remit $2.00 postage for the first book and 50¢ for each additional book.

Melvin Powers
12015 Sherman Road, No. Hollywood, California 91605

HOW TO GET RICH IN MAIL ORDER
by Melvin Powers

1. How to Develop Your Mail Order Expertise 2. How to Find a Unique Product or Service to Sell 3. How to Make Money with Classified Ads 4. How to Make Money with Display Ads 5. The Unlimited Potential for Making Money with Direct Mail 6. How to Copycat Successful Mail Order Operations 7. How I Created A Best Seller Using the Copycat Technique 8. How to Start and Run a Profitable Mail Order, Special Interest Book or Record Business 9. I Enjoy Selling Books by Mail — Some of My Successful and Not-So-Successful Ads and Direct Mail Circulars 10. Five of My Most Successful Direct Mail Pieces That Sold and Are Still Selling Millions of Dollars Worth of Books 11. Melvin Powers' Mail Order Success Strategy — Follow It and You'll Become a Millionaire 12. How to Sell Your Products to Mail Order Companies, Retail Outlets, Jobbers, and Fund Raisers for Maximum Distribution and Profits 13. How to Get Free Display Ads and Publicity That Can Put You on the Road to Riches 14. How to Make Your Advertising Copy Sizzle to Make You Wealthy 15. Questions and Answers to Help You Get Started Making Money in Your Own Mail Order Business 16. A Personal Word from Melvin Powers 17. How to Get Started Making Money in Mail Order. 18. Selling Products on Television - An Exciting Challenge   8½"x11" — 352 Pages...$20.00

HOW TO SELF-PUBLISH YOUR BOOK AND HAVE THE FUN AND EXCITEMENT OF BEING A BEST-SELLING AUTHOR
by Melvin Powers

An expert's step-by-step guide to marketing your book successfully 240 Pages...$20.00

A NEW GUIDE TO RATIONAL LIVING
by Albert Ellis, Ph.D. & Robert A. Harper, Ph.D.

1. How Far Can You Go With Self-Analysis? 2. You Feel the Way You Think 3. Feeling Well by Thinking Straight 4. How You Create Your Feelings 5. Thinking Yourself Out of Emotional Disturbances 6. Recognizing and Attacking Neurotic Behavior 7. Overcoming the Influences of the Past 8. Does Reason Always Prove Reasonable? 9. Refusing to Feel Desperately Unhappy 10. Tackling Dire Needs for Approval 11. Eradicating Dire Fears of Failure 12. How to Stop Blaming and Start Living 13. How to Feel Undepressed though Frustrated 14. Controlling Your Own Destiny 15. Conquering Anxiety   256 Pages...$7.00

PSYCHO-CYBERNETICS
A New Technique for Using Your Subconscious Power
by Maxwell Maltz, M.D., F.I.C.S.

1. The Self Image: Your Key to a Better Life 2. Discovering the Success Mechanism Within You 3. Imagination—The First Key to Your Success Mechanism 4. Dehypnotize Yourself from False Beliefs 5. How to Utilize the Power of Rational Thinking 6. Relax and Let Your Success Mechanism Work for You 7. You Can Acquire the Habit of Happiness 8. Ingredients of the Success-Type Personality and How to Acquire Them 9. The Failure Mechanism: How to Make It Work For You Instead of Against You 10. How to Remove Emotional Scars, or How to Give Yourself an Emotional Face Lift 11. How to Unlock Your Real Personality 12. Do-It-Yourself Tranquilizers   288 Pages...$7.00

A PRACTICAL GUIDE TO SELF-HYPNOSIS
by Melvin Powers

1. What You Should Know About Self-Hypnosis 2. What About the Dangers of Hypnosis? 3. Is Hypnosis the Answer? 4. How Does Self-Hypnosis Work? 5. How to Arouse Yourself from the Self-Hypnotic State 6. How to Attain Self-Hypnosis 7. Deepening the Self-Hypnotic State 8. What You Should Know About Becoming an Excellent Subject 9. Techniques for Reaching the Somnambulistic State 10. A New Approach to Self-Hypnosis When All Else Fails 11. Psychological Aids and Their Function 12. The Nature of Hypnosis 13. Practical Applications of Self-Hypnosis   144 Pages...$5.00

The books listed above can be obtained from your book dealer or directly from Melvin Powers. When ordering, please remit $2.00 postage for the first book and 50¢ for each additional book.

Melvin Powers
12015 Sherman Road, No. Hollywood, California 91605